# MAGICAL HEALING
## A HEALTH SURVIVAL GUIDE FOR OCCULTISTS, PAGANS, HEALERS, AND TAROT READERS

BY JOSEPHINE MCCARTHY

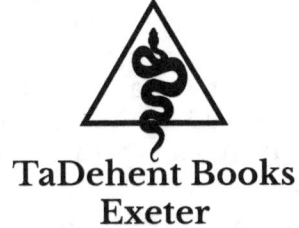

TaDehent Books
Exeter

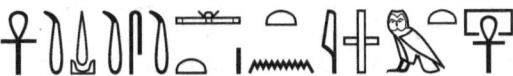

Copyright 2019 © Josephine McCarthy

All rights reserved

Without limiting the rights under copyright reserved above, no part of this publication may be reproduced, stored in, or introduced into a retrieval system, or transmitted, in any form or by any means (electronic, mechanical, photocopying, recording or otherwise) without prior permission of the copyright owner and the publisher of this book.

Originally published by Apocryphile Press USA

This edition published by:
TaDehent Books
Exeter UK
2019

ISBN 978-1-911134-38-1    hardback
ISBN 978-1-911134-40-4    paperback
ISBN 978-1-911134-39-8    ebook

Cover image by Stuart Littlejohn
Typeset by Michael Sheppard

**Disclaimer**
This book is intended to inform and compliment. It is not a replacement or alternative for medical treatment by a healthcare professional.
    The medical information in this book is not advice and should not be treated as such.
    You must not rely on the information in this book as an alternative to seeking medical advice from your doctor or other professional healthcare provider. If you have any specific questions about any medical matter, you should consult your doctor or other professional healthcare provider. If you think you may be suffering from any medical condition, you should seek immediate medical attention.
    You should never delay seeking medical advice, disregard medical advice or discontinue medical treatment because of information presented in this book.
    The author makes no representations or warranties in relation to the medical information presented in this book.

Dedicated to Stuart Littlejohn

and to Frater Acher,
for encouraging me to write this book

**Acknowledgements**
A massive thanks to the following people who, through their friendship, encouragement, advice, help, feedback and suggestions, enabled this book to come about:

Stuart Littlejohn, Frater Acher, Jon and Andrea, Toni, Tony, Christin, and finally to my daughters Cassandra and Leander for being such awesome, creative, clever and inspiring offspring.

# Contents

**Introduction**    1

**1 Knowing your body: part 1**    5
- 1.1 What you need to know about engines . . . . . . . . . . . 5
- 1.2 'Power in' . . . . . . . . . . . . . . . . . . . . . . . . . . . . 6
- 1.3 In the beginning . . . . . . . . . . . . . . . . . . . . . . . 7
- 1.4 Food and drink . . . . . . . . . . . . . . . . . . . . . . . . 8
- 1.5 Carbohydrates . . . . . . . . . . . . . . . . . . . . . . . . 9
- 1.6 Proteins . . . . . . . . . . . . . . . . . . . . . . . . . . . . 10
- 1.7 Drugs, medicines and alcohol . . . . . . . . . . . . . . . . 13
- 1.8 Antidepressants . . . . . . . . . . . . . . . . . . . . . . . . 14
- 1.9 Hypnotics, opiates, alcohol, THC and medical marijuana 17
- 1.10 Alcohol . . . . . . . . . . . . . . . . . . . . . . . . . . . . . 19
- 1.11 Visionary and hallucinogenic drugs . . . . . . . . . . . . 20
- 1.12 Chemical shit-storms . . . . . . . . . . . . . . . . . . . . . 23
- 1.13 Summary . . . . . . . . . . . . . . . . . . . . . . . . . . . 26

**2 Knowing your body: part 2**    29
- 2.1 Checks and balances: energy in, energy out . . . . . . . . 29
- 2.2 Living or working in a city . . . . . . . . . . . . . . . . . . 31
- 2.3 Empathy: other people and beings . . . . . . . . . . . . . 34
- 2.4 Inner alarms . . . . . . . . . . . . . . . . . . . . . . . . . . 35
- 2.5 Energetic boundaries . . . . . . . . . . . . . . . . . . . . . 36
- 2.6 Talismans . . . . . . . . . . . . . . . . . . . . . . . . . . . 39
- 2.7 Protecting and healing within your sphere . . . . . . . . 40
- 2.8 Sex . . . . . . . . . . . . . . . . . . . . . . . . . . . . . . . 41
- 2.9 Raising kids . . . . . . . . . . . . . . . . . . . . . . . . . . 42
- 2.10 Summary . . . . . . . . . . . . . . . . . . . . . . . . . . . 43

**3 Energy and magic**    45
- 3.1 Paying the piper: the price of advanced magic . . . . . . 45
- 3.2 Magic and energy . . . . . . . . . . . . . . . . . . . . . . . 46
- 3.3 Visionary and inner magic . . . . . . . . . . . . . . . . . . 46
- 3.4 Bridging . . . . . . . . . . . . . . . . . . . . . . . . . . . . 46
- 3.5 Inner study . . . . . . . . . . . . . . . . . . . . . . . . . . 48
- 3.6 Observing to bring change: magical exploration . . . . . 51
- 3.7 Power weaving . . . . . . . . . . . . . . . . . . . . . . . . 53

|  |  |  |
|---|---|---|
| 3.8 | Energetic consequences of working with deities | 54 |
| 3.9 | Conditional magic and body effects | 56 |
| 3.10 | Long-term projects | 58 |
| 3.11 | Ritualizing the action | 59 |
| 3.12 | Retirement: knowing when to back out | 60 |
| 3.13 | Summary | 61 |

## 4 Symptoms, reasons and power dynamics — 63
- 4.1 The reactor reaching critical mass .......... 63
- 4.2 Magical impacts .......... 64
- 4.3 Examples of impacts .......... 65
- 4.4 Magical imbalances .......... 68
- 4.5 Adrenals .......... 68
- 4.6 Thyroid .......... 72
- 4.7 Gland summary .......... 74
- 4.8 Magical catalysts .......... 75
- 4.9 Beings and the disturbance of the mind .......... 76
- 4.10 Intrusion .......... 76
- 4.11 Beings meet viruses in your body .......... 79

## 5 Tarot as a healing tool: layouts — 83
- 5.1 Peering through the looking glass .......... 83
- 5.2 Points to think about .......... 84
- 5.3 Layouts .......... 85
- 5.4 The health layout .......... 85
- 5.5 When to use the health layout .......... 92
- 5.6 The endocrine layout .......... 92
- 5.7 The four-directional layout: power incoming .......... 97
- 5.8 The Desert/Inner Landscape layout .......... 99
- 5.9 The Tree of Life layout .......... 102
- 5.10 Shuffling .......... 104
- 5.11 Cleaning hands and decks .......... 105
- 5.12 Summary .......... 106

## 6 Tarot as a healing tool: interpretation — 107
- 6.1 Reading the signs .......... 107
- 6.2 Diagnostic reading .......... 108
- 6.3 The last three years .......... 122
- 6.4 General interpretation advice .......... 126

## 7 Visionary healing: part one — 129
- 7.1 Going down the rabbit hole .......... 129
- 7.2 When to use visionary healing .......... 131
- 7.3 Stillness .......... 132
- 7.4 Cleaning and vacuuming, sewing and patching .......... 132
- 7.5 The guardians of the organs .......... 134
- 7.6 Colouring with the organs .......... 136

|       |                                                                  |     |
|-------|------------------------------------------------------------------|-----|
| 7.7   | Working with the endocrine system                                | 137 |
| 7.8   | The inner landscape                                              | 139 |
| 7.9   | Working with the patterns of life force                          | 142 |
| 7.10  | Summary                                                          | 144 |

## 8 Visionary healing: part two — 147
| | | |
|---|---|---|
| 8.1 | The call for help | 147 |
| 8.2 | Working with Sekhmet | 148 |
| 8.3 | Vision of Sekhmet | 149 |
| 8.4 | Repairing the pattern | 152 |
| 8.5 | Finding the right realm and contacts for the job | 154 |
| 8.6 | Approaching a contact for healing | 155 |
| 8.7 | Summary | 156 |

## 9 Homeopathy — 157
| | | |
|---|---|---|
| 9.1 | Little pills that pack a punch | 157 |
| 9.2 | Key remedies | 159 |
| 9.3 | *Aconitum napellus* (Monkshood) | 160 |
| 9.4 | *Arnica* (Arnica montana) | 160 |
| 9.5 | *Arsenicum album* | 160 |
| 9.6 | *Hypericum perforatum* (St. Johns wort) | 161 |
| 9.7 | *Gelsemium* | 162 |
| 9.8 | Nitric acid | 162 |
| 9.9 | Sulphur | 163 |
| 9.10 | How to take homeopathic remedies (and how to store them) | 163 |
| 9.11 | Choosing the right potency | 164 |
| 9.12 | How remedies work and what to expect | 165 |
| 9.13 | Demons/disease consciousness and nosodes | 167 |
| 9.14 | Summary | 169 |

## 10 Herbs and Substances — 171
| | | |
|---|---|---|
| 10.1 | Just a spoonful of sugar | 171 |
| 10.2 | Head and brain | 172 |
| 10.3 | Heart impact | 174 |
| 10.4 | Bone, joint and muscle injuries | 175 |
| 10.5 | Skin neuralgia | 176 |
| 10.6 | Burns | 176 |
| 10.7 | Endocrine imbalances and the menopause | 177 |
| 10.8 | St. Johns wort (*Hypericum perforatum*) | 179 |
| 10.9 | Siberian Ginseng (*Eleutherococcus senticosus*) | 180 |
| 10.10 | Kelp (*Laminaria*) | 180 |
| 10.11 | Velvet bean (*Mucuna pruriens*) | 181 |
| 10.12 | Shatavari (*Asparagus racemosus*) | 181 |
| 10.13 | Ashwagandha (*Withania somnifera*) | 181 |
| 10.14 | Chamomile (*Matricaria chamomilla, Chamaemelum nobile*) | 182 |
| 10.15 | Anti-inflammatory herbs | 182 |

|     | 10.16 | Protective herbs for the land | 183 |
| --- | --- | --- | --- |
|     | 10.17 | Useful garden herbs for magic or medicine | 184 |
|     | 10.18 | Using your own herbs | 186 |
|     | 10.19 | House protection: making bundles | 186 |
|     | 10.20 | Infusions | 187 |
|     | 10.21 | Tinctures | 187 |
|     | 10.22 | Poultice | 188 |
|     | 10.23 | Summary | 189 |
| **11** | **Approaches to self-healing and maintenance** | | **191** |
|     | 11.1 | Magical, emotional, and physical considerations | 191 |
|     | 11.2 | Emotional baggage | 191 |
|     | 11.3 | Magical maintenance | 193 |
|     | 11.4 | Keeping clear of tangles | 194 |
|     | 11.5 | Everything has its own time for resolution | 197 |
|     | 11.6 | Energetic resources | 198 |
|     | 11.7 | Scapegoating | 201 |
|     | 11.8 | Physical maintenance | 203 |
|     | 11.9 | Getting maintenance work done | 203 |
|     | 11.10 | Astrology | 204 |
|     | 11.11 | Lose the New Age bullshit | 205 |
|     | 11.12 | Summary | 206 |
| **A** | **The ritual cleansing of a space, room, or house** | | **207** |
|     | A.1 | Recitation for the consecration of salt and water | 207 |
|     | A.2 | Recitation of pouring | 208 |
|     | A.3 | Cleansing a space | 208 |
|     | A.4 | Recitation of clearing | 209 |
|     | A.5 | Ritual bath for body cleansing | 209 |
| **B** | **Technique for making a talisman** | | **211** |
|     | B.1 | Setting up | 211 |
|     | B.2 | Creating the talisman | 212 |
|     | B.3 | Maintenance | 213 |
| **C** | **Tarot key words for health readings** | | **215** |
|     | C.1 | The Minor Arcana | 216 |
|     | C.2 | The Major Arcana: the trump cards | 218 |

# *Introduction*

When I wrote the book *The Magic of the North Gate*, I started to broach the subject of the relationship between the body and magic. I offered general advice to the magician, along with various methods and techniques for tending to the magician's body. Since that time, I have been swamped with letters, emails and requests for a more in-depth look at the issues surrounding a magician and his or her health—hence this book.

Throughout these chapters we will look at the relationship between magic and bodily health, and how the path of magic and the path of body awareness are inextricably linked. We will also look at specific healing modalities, magical impacts on health, consciousness of the body and techniques to maintain body strength. The techniques, ideas and suggestions presented in this book are designed to support you in your magical practice and also to compliment your regular health care provided by your doctor.

When I began to work more powerfully within the sphere of magic I became aware of my body and how it struggled against the strains I was inflicting upon it. I was also aware of how magic strengthened many things within me; a bittersweet relationship. That set me upon a road of deep discovery in terms of magic and the body, which eventually led me to realize that many prominent magicians in the past had also made this powerful connection between magic, body and health. Dion Fortune and her partner Dr Penry Evans were fascinated by this weave of power between body and magic, and Franz Bardon, the Czech adept, also understood the necessity for healing, magic and energetic body awareness to go hand in hand.

In today's world where everything is compartmentalized, this wisdom of the need for a wide breadth of knowledge in the magician is sadly falling by the wayside. Every magician who works with power will come up against a barrier of body and health issues at some point. Hopefully this book will help the magician make solid choices and become responsible for

# Introduction

their own energy, health and wellbeing. It will also expose the harsh truth that magic can be a struggle for both body and soul. In today's bullshit world of the New Age movement where everything is always light, fluffy and glowing with health, a reality check is sorely needed.

It is also worth mentioning at this point that I am neither a doctor, nor a qualified health professional. A qualified doctor or health professional should always be your first port of call if you become sick.

The information provided in this book comes from direct experience gained from experimentation, informal study with health professionals, my own educational background, and years of learning, trial and error. I have struggled with a variety of health issues over the years; some are genetic or inherited illnesses, some are the direct result of magic (and my own stupidity), and some were matters of circumstance, accident and disease. Throughout all of these I have endeavoured to find my own solutions where I could, develop my own coping mechanisms, and to learn as much as I can.

This book is the result of my successes and failures. I write it for those coming up behind me on the magical ladder of learning as well as those alongside me who missed this rung. Truly, if I had this book in my hands when I was in my twenties and thirties, I would have avoided a lot of suffering and struggle. If I can help other magicians avoid that same struggle, even in the smallest way, then this book will have been time well spent.

Many young magicians never give their bodies a second thought. In their twenties they are full of vitality, health and vigour; health is something for the doctor to worry about as they scour the latest goatskin-bound grimoire looking for another obscure ritual to inflict upon the world. And for many, that total disconnect will continue throughout their adult lives until they hit their forties or fifties, at which point things begin to go badly wrong.

Some magicians become aware early on that the more powerful the magic the bigger the impact on the body, yet they will still ignore the warning signs that their body desperately sends out. A few will get the message and begin to look for ways to maintain their bodies, to lessen impacts, and to treat the body with more respect when it does succumb to illnesses or injuries.

This is not a medical or 'health' guide book. Rather, it is a magical approach to health, disease and injury, and it exposes the many interconnected dynamics between the body, soul, energy and magic that we so often blithely ignore.

Our bodies and their reactions are truly unique. While some illnesses have specific symptomatic patterns, others do not and these continue to confound doctors. When you do magic, particularly visionary magic, the symptomatic picture that the body presents when ill often changes: the body shifts how it responds to invaders, imbalances and impacts. Magic does not make you sick *per se*, but not tending to your body and not approaching your magic wisely can eventually make you weak and ill.

So if you are intent on delving deeper and deeper into magic or you are already there up to your knees in power and sporting a really bad headache, it might be worth taking the time to learn more about the body's relationship with magic. To do that, you need to know your own body, how it functions and how it reacts. It is not necessary to learn full human biology, anatomy and physiology etc, but if you do have those under your belt then they will be useful. I learned these subjects in my late teens and early twenties as part of my training to become a ballet teacher. It served me well in ballet, but even better in magic!

If you want to flourish as an adept it is important to learn a good solid healing modality—and more than one if possible. Through learning a specific form of healing you will also learn about the body and the various ways of approaching its care and upkeep. Taking the time to study, experiment and practise a healing modality not only serves you as a magician, it also serves those around you.

Do not take the advice in this book as an alternative to seeking out medical help: often we need the care and expertise that the medical profession can offer us. Rather, approach this book as a resource that a magician can use to actively engage in their own healing alongside allopathic medical treatment.

It has become fashionable in magical circles to reject all that medicine has to offer: that is true folly. Mainstream medicine does not have all the answers and probably never will, but it does have some pretty awesome aspects and can come in very handy. There are times for mainstream medicine, times for alternative healing and times to use both. Without mainstream medicine, I would not be alive to write this book. In fact I would not have written any books: since my childhood a combination of surgery, medicines and medical care has kept me alive and

## Introduction

on my feet. Without hospitals I would have died at the age of ten when my appendix ruptured.

Similarly when I contracted Scarlet Fever, without antibiotic treatment I would not have survived. Throughout my life I have struggled with many illnesses and accidents that have taken me close to death. Many of them were treated with mainstream medicine along with alternative treatments to patch me up afterwards.

On the other hand, magical techniques and alternative therapies have saved my ass when medicine could not. So the moral of the story, and the purpose of this book, is to give you a wider and more grounded understanding of how to navigate through your magical life in a flexible, intelligent and informed way. Magic in its full power changes the goal posts when it comes to our bodies, and a major skill in magic is to know how to react and adapt when your body is under strain.

Do not shun any healing possibility out of an ignorant following of current popular opinion. Nor is it wise to follow any 'magic cure' out of faith, wishful thinking or new age glamour. Educate yourself. Learn how your own body works, and which energy dynamics in magic affect you and which do not. And most importantly of all, listen to your body, use your common sense and take responsibility for yourself.

Chapter One

# *Knowing your body: part 1*

## 1.1  What you need to know about engines

As a magician, your greatest and most precious tool is your own body. If this does not operate properly or is uncared for, then your magic has no foundation to rest upon. The more power you work with, the more important it is to respect your body and attend properly to its needs.

Studying detailed human biology is not necessary, but knowing how your body works in simple terms is very important. You need to know how it processes energy, how its structure is upheld, and how it regulates itself.

'Power in,' 'power maintained' and 'power out'—those are the first basics of which you need a rudimentary understanding. 'Power in' is the diet, all incoming energies, and all emotions. 'Power maintained' is the job of the endocrine system, a delicate structure that is often disrupted by magic. 'Power out' is what is expressed through the digestive system, skin, fluids and magical actions.

These are all directly affected for both good and bad by magic; hence it is important to understand them. But remember, the combination of an individual and a specific path of magic makes for a unique picture; there is no 'one size fits all' or 'one pill heals all' scenario.

The path of tending to a magical body is a major stream of magical learning all of itself, so do not neglect it or consider it to be something that is solved with a herbal pill each morning. The body and its reactions to magical work will teach you more about magical power than any fancy grimoire can.

So let's look at a few basic mechanics. We will start with 'power in,' which is essentially anything that goes into your mouth, is put on your skin, or passes into your system via magic. The first 'power in' on that list is the one that is most overlooked: what goes into your mouth. People will talk about magical alchemy

# 1. Knowing your body: part 1

in reverent whispers but never give much thought to what they put into their mouths.

When you practise magic, what you put into your body can often have a much more reactive effect than normal and the more powerful the magic, the more of a reaction you will potentially experience. Many magicians report this phenomenon when they achieve powerful levels of working, and yet few think sensibly about it. Many find they are forced to alter their diets or lifestyles, or to give up certain foods or substances, or to otherwise change their relationship with what they put in their mouths or on their bodies.

## 1.2 'Power in'

*Food, drink, drugs, sex, magical contact and smelly perfumes*

The 'power in' list is one that triggers all sorts of arrogant posturing from soap boxes. There are people who get all evangelical about a diet, a drug, a secret contact or a magical oil. But wherever there is a wonder drug or a special magical substance to be had, there is usually also a price tag, often high, that someone wants you to pay. Whenever the loud posturing is about abstinence, there is often an ego or messiah complex lurking in the background.

Any restriction or issue with a 'power in' substance should be about your individual body and its relationship to a specific magical form—it is about what the body needs and what it does not need. Morals, status or beliefs should have nothing to do with it. Magic does not need a soap box; it needs a tool box, and one that works well.

Sometimes a restriction or an altered body response is directly connected to a deity or a particular line of magical work; in such cases it is wise to take things a step at a time and be willing to be flexible. Often this sort of 'power in' issue is specific to a particular frequency of magical power and once that work is finished then the issue fades away. There will be times when a deity asks you not to eat, drink or partake of certain substances. Again this is not to do with morality; it is most often connected to how their power works in relation to human bodies. Let us look into the background of some of these issues, and how it is best to approach them in order to uphold the magical body.

## 1.3 In the beginning

The societal changes in the Western world that have happened over the last hundred or so years have also brought with them subsequent health issues, and many of those issues trace back to diet. Food has moved from being a necessary fuel to being a pastime, a drug, and a substance of indulgence. This is not a new thing for humanity, but it has become far more widespread and normalized since the industrial revolution, before which it was a preserve only of the rich and powerful. Add to that the way food has been chemically and genetically modified over the last few decades, and we have a potential health time-bomb waiting to go off.

Most babies these days are bottle-fed from birth. They are given weaning foods very early on, and are introduced to chemicals and foods long before their bodies are ready to cope with them. As a net result, babies who are sensitive or have inherited a tendency to develop autoimmune issues are being groomed for a life of ill health from birth. Dairy and grains are both major triggers for intestinal imbalances in vulnerable babies, as is the modern lack of bacterial exposure during birth which would normally prime the infant's immune system and digestion in a balanced way. What has this got to do with magic? Everything.

When a magician begins to work with inner or ritual power, the body will make use of that inflow of power to address its own problems. That is the first issue. The second issue is that when power and beings flow from the inner worlds to the outer worlds and pass through or around the magician, the immune system will see them as potential invaders, and this often sets off a small immune reaction.

If the magician has any underlying problems with their immune system these will be triggered, and that will create a series of reactions in the body. Stillness/void meditation and yoga are two things that will help to lessen this reaction and allow the body to get used to such power without reacting as if it is under attack.

But if the magician was exposed as a baby to foods that affected their intestinal bacteria and immune responses, then that pattern of reaction will already be deeply embedded in their body. The result will be an 'inflammatory flare' within the magician. The older the magician, the more likely such a flare will occur.

# 1. Knowing your body: part 1

This very early exposure to dairy and grains is important to keep in mind when looking for healing and stabilizing modalities as a magical tool. The more potential for magic a person is born with, the more there is potential for their body to be sensitive and reactive.

Some of the most useful healing and health support modalities that a magician can use (for example Chinese medicine, homeopathy and herbs) work from the premise that their patient was breast-fed, and usually exclusively for at least the first year of their life. That is often no longer the case. We are living in a world where a new baby is immediately exposed to substances, chemicals, vaccines and foods that its little body was not designed to cope with. This deep shift is changing how our immune systems operate; in turn we must adapt how we treat our bodies.

So if you are a practitioner of acupuncture, herbs, homeopathy etc, it is helpful to understand that what would have easily rebalanced someone one hundred years ago will not work in quite the same way today. You do not need to abandon the healing modality, but it is wise to understand that some people's systems have been damaged from birth and their immune systems have adapted around that. To compensate, the treatments also need to adapt. You may not always be able to arrive at a still point of health, but you can help the altered body to be the best that it possibly can be within the circumstances.

The first step in supporting a modern body is to pay attention to its unique nutritional needs. There are many books, blogs and courses that teach fad diets or have general food advice. The one fall-down is that no two bodies are exactly alike, and this is particularly true of magical bodies. The more you work with magic, the more unique your body's needs become. The key is learning to listen to your body, to observe, to pay attention and to use your common sense. But there are some general snippets of information regarding magic and food that can be useful. The following section is based upon my own personal experiences (which may be very different to yours) and from treating other magicians over long periods of time.

## 1.4   Food and drink

The first thing to be aware of is that the body is constantly changing and renewing itself. A person's immune system shifts and changes over the years, and for a magician that will be all the more apparent. So what will be fine for you in your twenties will not be fine in your late thirties or forties. Things that were not good for your body in your thirties become fine in your fifties... And so on. The key to working with fluctuating patterns like these is the same valuable key we find everywhere in magic: pay attention. Nothing stays the same: the body and mind are immensely dynamic and you truly have to be on the ball to keep up with them. And remember, the more you are involved in magic, the more dynamic the changes become. Let's look first at the foods that create the most reactions, for both good and bad.

## 1.5 Carbohydrates

Carbs are your fuel. When you have finished a round of heavy magic, the first thing the body screams for is fuel. A wise magician neither fully indulges the body nor starves it after a magical working: either response will prime the body for problems. The fuel intake needs to be enough to ground the magician and replenish their body's stores of energy without overfeeding it.

In truth, the body is screaming for inner as well as outer energy, so you must attend to both rather than giving it only one fuel source. Inner regeneration comes from sleep, meditation, and from cutting all inner contact. That is easily achieved by doing something which has no inner interaction: something that is passive like watching TV or reading a trashy (non-magical) novel or best of all going for a walk in nature or simply lying in the garden.

The outer fuel should be a light intake of carbohydrate. This is where the first hurdle of immune response should be addressed. Certain carbohydrates will trigger an immune response in a body that has been primed from youth to react to them. The biggest culprit, for those who are sensitive, is grains. If you are not sensitive, then any good quality organic grain will suffice. If you are unfortunate enough to be grain- or gluten-sensitive, then look to root carbs like potatoes. And I mean real potatoes, not the reconstituted mush reshaped into fries and sold in frozen packs or at fast food outlets.

How do you know if you are sensitive to grains? Do you have digestion problems? IBS? Do you have low or high abdominal pain a couple of hours after eating? Do you get brain fog after eating? An easy way to check (and I use the word 'easy' in the

## 1. Knowing your body: part 1

loosest possible sense) is to stop eating all grains for a couple of months. If your symptoms settle down, then grains or gluten were at the root of the issue. Reintroducing non-gluten grains first will either confirm or rule out gluten sensitivity. Grains and derivative substances are used to thicken everything from yogurt to stock cubes, so if you are grain-sensitive, you will need to read the labels.

The key is to pay attention, listen to your body and have enough self-discipline to be able to stop eating or drinking something that is ultimately poisonous to your specific body. Discipline is all part of the magical path.

Sugar is a substance that also gets lumped in under the heading of carbohydrates, but it is processed in a slightly different way by the body. It has become the evil aunt of the food groups, but ordinary sugar (the best is unrefined molasses sugar) is of no real harm unless you are well on your way to becoming diabetic, or you also eat a lot of carbs. The body needs a chunk of sugar each day to keep the brain ticking over, most of which it gains from the eating of grains, roots, fruits, and veggies. Sugar in sensible amounts is not evil, and there have been times when my body has really needed it after a heavy round of magic. Like all these things, you have to listen to your body and use your common sense, as everyone is slightly different.

### 1.6 Proteins

The way we gain our protein is an issue that is heavily entwined with religious and magical thinking. Some paths and religions demand we eat no animal flesh; others have particular meats that are taboo. These restrictions are often connected either with the worship of a specific deity or philosophy, or to the genetic health issues of a particular group of people.

If you choose to be vegetarian for ethical or health reasons, then it is important to be aware that certain types of magical work will be much harder on your body, and also that certain streams of magic will be far more accessible to you. Depending on how your individual body copes with a meat-free diet, it would be wise to pay very close attention to which areas of magical practice impact you the most, and either avoid them or work around them.

Similarly if you are not willing to go without meat for certain lengths of time, other areas of magic will be limited for you or may be difficult or dangerous to practise. To operate in a

## 1.6. Proteins

wide spectrum of magic requires mutability and a willingness to adapt—that is the first and most important key to staying in one piece over many years of working in the magical inner worlds.

I have been vegan, vegetarian and carnivore, and each switch in my diet was due to my magical practice and health. It also seemed to have a strong correlation to the land power of the specific area where I was living at the time.

The first thing you should do around the protein issue is to step back from all the philosophies and taboos and look at it from your perspective as a magician. The questions you need to ask yourself are: What does your body need (rather than want)? What demands do magical acts put on your particular body? What land are you living on and what are the land spirits like? What deity are you working with? And finally, what specific inner realms are you working with magically? Let's look at these questions one at a time.

Some bodies do not do well with meat. Some do not do well without meat. And there is a whole range of in-betweens. It is important to know your own body, and how it reacts to things. Those reactions will come from a variety of sources: your genetic make up, your childhood upbringing, the land you live on, any conditions you have, etc. Finding out how your body operates normally, outside of magic, will give you a baseline from which you will be able to understand better the various strains and impacts that different types of magic have on your body. The differences are most obvious when it comes to protein intake.

One word of practical caution though – if you are vegan or spending some time being vegan, ensure that you have a full intake of the recommended daily amount of iodine (usually through vegan vitamins). In the USA the salt has added iodine, so it is not so much of an issue. But in other countries a vegan has no source of iodine, and iodine keeps the thyroid functioning normally. Magicians often put their thyroids under strain with magic, so it is wise to ensure you get a proper dose each day (and no more than the daily recommended amount of 150mcg).

It is important to understand that religions and philosophies that practise vegetarianism often originated in warm countries where lots of non-animal protein sources were readily available, whereas religions that include meat as a part of their pattern often emerged out of colder climates. We are more racially mixed than our ancestors, we have a wealth of food available,

## 1. Knowing your body: part 1

and we are more mobile, so climate and food source availability are not such issues for us.

But the inherited resonances are still within us and they need to be taken into consideration. Some body types just do not do well with certain types of protein, whereas others can eat anything that runs. Find out which proteins feed you and which do not—it is that simple. Forget any other consideration at this point: it is important to know what your needs are so that you can work around them if you have to, such as having to switch diets for magical reasons.

The land that you live on is a major component in the decision of what to eat and what not to eat. As a magician, the land you live on, the land you do magic on, and the land beings that are around you all have a direct influence on what you should eat. The reasons for this are many and varied.

Over the years I have noticed that eating meat on certain lands is needful, whereas when living in other areas eating meat or certain meats causes aggravation. Some land beings cannot see you if you do not eat meat and others will not go near you if you do. Some inner realms are more easily accessed and worked with if you are vegan; other inner realms are downright dangerous if you are not grounded with meat. Over the years I have changed diets back and forth according to what land I lived on, what magical work I was doing, and so forth.

As a magician it is wise to be willing to bend and flex, to be mutable and not to cling to philosophies or ways of thinking that are inappropriate for the path you are walking through life. The key is always within yourself, not in any outside information: your body will tell you if you listen to it.

Sometimes you will find that your body tunes in to a specific magical or religious taboo that involves food, particularly if you are working within a specific religious or magical stream. For example, I cannot eat pork. It makes me sick and makes me feel strange. I do not know why, only that it does. Similarly I cannot eat shellfish—actually I cannot stand even to be around shellfish, I find it repulsive. I do not eat diary, so I do not mix dairy and meats. I had not really thought about this (because I can be incredibly dumb at times) until a Rabbi friend of mine jokingly pointed out that I lived closer to Kosher than some of his family. Whether that is connected with my work in Kabbalah or it is just a coincidence, I don't know.

The more you listen to your body, the more you will hear it speak. If something makes you feel ill, do not immediately reach for the drugs; instead listen to what your body is trying to say to you and find out what is upsetting it.

Specific deities and their demands are another major component in the protein issue. In magic we do not worship a deity; that is the role of religion, not magic. But we do work respectfully with them, sometimes exclusively and intensely. In that tight working relationship, there is sometimes a need to adjust the diet in order to work in more depth with a specific deity power. The reasons for these dietary restrictions or additions has very much to do with how the power of that deity operates, and how your body's energy dovetails with theirs to create a harmonic and balanced power grid that can then be worked with. Sometimes you may well face restrictions that have little to do with any known taboos in connection to that deity; they could instead be specifically related to your body, the land you live on, and how your power operates in conjunction with the deity.

So for example, during the many years I spent working with the goddesses Kali and Durga, I could not eat any animal substance. Once that round of work was over, I was able to eat meat again. Do not assume that what books say about a deity and diet restrictions will be true for you: you must discover for yourself what the appropriate dietary and power relationship is between you and the powers with which you are working. But on the other hand, if the deity demands you become vegetarian while you work with them, and you ignore it and convince yourself it does not apply to you, then you may be in for a major body shock. I can tell you that sometimes these restrictions, be they traditional or individual to you, are there for a damn good reason and it has to do with your body's integrity within the sphere of magic.

## 1.7 Drugs, medicines and alcohol

Any substance that affects your consciousness, your brain, or your body's energy processing system is going to affect how you operate within magic, sometimes for the better and sometimes for the worse. Your body is a filter for magical power, so any issues with that filter are going to affect both the flow of magic and the integrity of the body it passes through.

The first key is to understand how these substances act within the body and how that interaction in turn affects magic. It is also very important to understand how certain beings involved in the flow of power and magic can potentially interact with your body and access your stores of energy when your filters are out of balance.

These substances are entangled with major controversies in our societies, and arguments are constantly being bandied back and forth about ethics versus freedom of choice, and individual versus collective health. However, the wider debate regarding the use of these substances is of no individual concern to the magician: how your body reacts and how your magic works is what is important.

The following list explores different types of substances and the possible effects they may have on your body, your magical actions, and the subsequent interactions with the beings around you. We will also look at reasons for taking these substances, and how those reasons can have a direct affect upon the magicians' life and work.

If a magician finds that they have to take a certain substance, for whatever reason, then it is important to know how it could affect their work and their body, and how to change their practice to accommodate its effects.

## 1.8 Antidepressants

Drugs that alter the level and uptake of serotonin in the body are prescribed for a variety of reasons, not just for depression. Magic uses serotonin as a buffer, or I should say, the body uses serotonin, dopamine and adrenaline to protect itself against magical impact during heavy work, hence the serotonin (and dopamine) 'high' when the inner gates open and the magical work is about to commence.

The human body's neurotransmitter chemistry works rather like a team of a million skilled jugglers all taking part in one mass, interlinked juggle. If just one of them goes out of sync, the whole show will begin to spin out of control. These chemicals are found not just in our brain but throughout our bodies, and they are engaged in a very delicate act of 'keeping balance.' Some neurotransmitters have a wide-reaching effect within the body and some have very specific actions. It does not take much to knock something out of balance.

If a person is depressed, they are prescribed antidepressants. The jugglers are out of balance for some reason: adding magic into that juggling act can help or hinder the rebalancing process

## 1.8. Antidepressants

depending on the cause of the depression, the way the magician copes with it and the medications that are prescribed.

Everyone gets depressed at some point in their life. But if someone has repeated long-term bouts of depression (bipolar disorder, for example) then their body will not be able to withstand powerful visionary magic, and in fact such magic would aggravate their condition, often to the point of psychosis.

Knowing that there are times when your body will need time out from magic is an important factor in keeping your body strong. If you have been suffering a bout of depression and you are taking antidepressants, then choose to work *with* your body magically, not against it. You can help the antidepressant and speed up the healing process by focusing on stillness meditation and working with the void in meditation, but nothing more than that in a visionary sense. Any other magical acts should be externalized ritual actions only, and even those should be simple maintenance rituals which do not involve any inner beings.

Some people need to take long term anti-depressants, usually because their own uptake mechanism is lacking something, or they produce too many receptors which means their body is in a constant struggle to produce the necessary serotonin for so many receptors. In such a case, once the person is stable, the medication should not have any adverse effect on their magic, and their magic should not affect them badly. Again, it always goes back to the individual – simply pay attention to your body and do what is right for you as an individual.

Remember that addressing depression is a time of healing, not of learning or work. Any magical work should be about healing and nothing more. Any ritual undertaken should just be about acknowledging the powers around you, tending deities or tending an altar: you are essentially treading water. Working with any beings, action rituals or visions at a vulnerable time like this will only weaken you more in the long term.

A positive way to be useful magically at such a time is to use your hands to make things, or organize things. Creating magical tools, paintings, icons, or shrines are outer magical actions that engage the creative process, which in turn helps the brain to engage its own healing abilities. For a magician, this is also a form of passive mediation. You are still bridging the worlds magically, but because you are not 'working' magically you tap into the inner stream of creative and regenerative power; power which will pass into your body before it goes into whatever it is you are making.

## 1. Knowing your body: part 1

The way to do this is very simple: no magical preparation, no use of sigils, visions, utterances, nothing. Simply begin making whatever it is you are going to make with a clear intent: I am going to make a magical wand, I am going to paint whatever needs painting, etc. It does not matter how it turns out, just let it be itself. Engaging that process will speed up your healing time and you will find that your need for the antidepressant slowly drops as your body begins to regain its sense of balance.

If you insist on doing magic while depressed and on antidepressants (or herbs) the magical action will burn up what available serotonin you have, which can result in a depressive crash the day after—with an added side-order of badly aching muscles and sleep disturbances. Depending on how depleted your body is, that crash could last days or months.

The neurotransmitter dopamine is also tied in with this magical dynamic of boom and bust. When the dopamine has also been burned up and the body is depleted through magic, the magician will develop restless legs, tremors, an out of sync body clock and emotional numbness. Learn to recognize these symptoms of burnout and if any of them appear in your life, it is time to step back from magic and take time out for the body to do its healing.

There is another form of depression which has implications for magicians, and that is the type that is linked to oestrogen and testosterone levels. In late teens until about thirty years old, and later in women, the hormones are at their peak. This can give a magician access to large amounts of power if they know what they are doing. Thankfully, 99.9% of magicians below the age of thirty-five do not really know how to tap into that power in any great depth, though a hormone-inflated ego may think differently.

You will probably have reached your forties before you really learn how to connect with and handle very deep inner power, by which time your body's outer capacity to match that power will have waned. This is a natural mechanism put in place to protect the rest of the world from your own rampant stupidity.

For those of you who are reading this and are in their forties or older, look back to when you were in your twenties. Can you remember how dumb you were, magically and emotionally? How even though you thought you were wise and knowledgeable, mature and grounded, you were actually an immature idiot? I know I was. Can you remember how much emotional power you had? Surges of anger, happiness, arousal, depression—that age-group gets the full stew. Add powerful magic to the mix and watch the bombs go off!

So if you are in that age group and you are suffering from depression as well as the hormone-fuelled wild ride, remember this: it is a harsh but normal phase of life in natural magicians. Use the hormonal power to learn how to operate your body. Give it physical exercise and discipline. This will in turn get you ready to operate the power you potentially could access later in life.

The depression will lift if you put the hormonal fuel to work: dance, martial arts, sports, or hard physical labour. That in turn will get your body ready to handle magical power. A powerful, strong body can take vast amounts of inner power flowing through it. An undernourished or weakly-developed body cannot.

## 1.9 Hypnotics, opiates, alcohol, THC and medical marijuana

There will come a time in most magicians' lives when they will use these substances for one reason or another, be it surgery, stress, pain, curiosity, recreation, etc. From a magical perspective it is wise to know that the majority of magicians find these substances lower their ability to mediate power or to handle power. They also loosen the inner boundaries which are there to guide you in visionary work.

That said, with long-term use the body and spirit can learn to adjust around some of these substances, but that long-term application brings with it a whole bag of other problems for the body and spirit. If you are on one of these substances for the long term and you wish to continue visionary magic then there are a few things you should consider.

The first is that any magical work should be done when the substance is least in your system, which means just before the next dose is due.

The second thing to consider is that if you are a long-term user of one of these substances, then it is either because of addiction, illness or injury. If you have any of these conditions, then deep work in the inner worlds will only aggravate them. Working deeply in magical vision involves having large amounts of power flowing through your body, and if that body is ill or broken in some way, it is a cracked vessel as far as many types of inner power are concerned. Cracked vessels leak and fall apart;

# 1. Knowing your body: part 1

that is essentially what happens when magicians mix these types of substances with deeper work. It puts a terrible strain on your body, so keep that in mind.

Under such circumstances it is better to shift the working practice to more externalized and naturally-formed non-visionary magic. Visionary work can still be done, but it is best done very rarely, simply, and using well-trodden paths to places in the inner worlds that you know to be safe. The key is only to do what really needs doing, not what you want to do: spend the time learning and consolidating.

Be very aware that if you are on these substances, your focus is likely to be impaired and your boundaries weak, which in turn can make you vulnerable. Many magicians find that when they take such substances the visionary process will just not work. If that happens, do not fight it: it is your body's defence system kicking in to block you out of the inner worlds for your own protection. Listen to your body; it will guide you.

It can be very frustrating for a magician who wishes to work deeply in magic but also has to take medication which disrupts the process; it is wise to think very carefully about what you do to your body and mind. Here is a classic example of how these substances can affect a magician.

A couple of years ago, I had major surgery and was on morphine for quite some time. Morphine in particular can loosen the bond between a person's body and spirit in a potentially dangerous way, and particularly if that person is a visionary magician, for in such cases that bond is already fluid. While I was on morphine I did no magic at all, but every night when I was asleep I turned up in the dreams of my old students, and gave lectures on magical technique. I was completely unaware of this and only found out about it when these former students individually emailed me. Every morning I would wake up exhausted and weak, and my life force was already at a very low ebb from the surgery.

Once I had figured out what I was doing and where my energy was going, I made a talisman to 'lock' my spirit into my body so it could not go wandering off lecturing people every night. I also realized that if my own natural boundaries had become a lot more porous and I was 'leaking out,' then I was also vulnerable to lots of predatory beings who could potentially feed off of my life force.

I set up guardians to watch over my body and put on the locking talisman, and hey presto! the visits stopped, and I started to recover. I began to get stronger, to heal faster and to get my energy back. I guess because I was so ill, my spirit felt that I had to pass on as much as I could before I died. That is a natural reaction to a threat to one's life, but it can also speed up the dying process as it uses so much inner energy.

If similar things happen to you, rather than thinking it cool and leaving it at that, think very carefully about the consequences of such behaviour for your life force. If you are a visionary magician, then any drug that sends you into a deep uncontrolled sleep or otherwise dampens your consciousness can put you at risk.

## 1.10 Alcohol

Alcohol is in a class of its own when it comes to substances that affect magic. Alcohol has a major dampening affect on your inner boundaries, and leaves you wide open to all sorts of beings taking up residence in your space. Some magicians use it to cut a contact or to dampen down inner sight. It does both those things very effectively, but in more than very small quantities is also leaves you very vulnerable. This is the key reason why many visionary magicians find that the deeper they work in vision, the less tolerance they have for alcohol.

If you find your alcohol tolerance begins to lower (and you are not an alcoholic – lowered tolerance can also be a symptom of physical dependency), then take it as a signal from your body that your defences are going down. Under such circumstances it is wise to stop using alcohol at all.

I cannot drink more that a few mouthfuls before I feel my barriers crumbling and my inner senses decaying. In my teens I used to drink a lot, as it blocked out my ability to 'see' spirits and pick up on subtle energies. I wanted a quiet life, and I did not have the magical knowledge at that time to cope with such contact.

Eventually I realized that by shutting down my senses, I was putting myself in danger and making myself vulnerable. I stopped drinking and within a few months crossed paths with my first teacher who showed me how to handle my senses properly and to work with them magically. I had made a decision to stop hiding, and the inner worlds responded to that decision by guiding me towards someone who could help me develop and grow.

# 1. Knowing your body: part 1

## 1.11 Visionary and hallucinogenic drugs

There is a lot of discussion in magical circles about the use of visionary drugs as a tool in magic. Most of this stems from Western interest in the use of hallucinogenic substances in tribal magic, and from the use of LSD. There are a few things to consider here when it comes to visionary magic.

The first is that if you are trying to work with visionary magic, then using these substances will degrade your work considerably. Why? Because visionary magic is about the conscious use of a technique that, when developed and applied, allows you to pass between the different inner and outer realms in a controlled and focused manner. Anything that removes that focus and control is contraindicated.

There are no shortcuts to developing visionary skills, and the use of these substances bypasses all structures, guardians and boundaries that are in place not only to guide you through the inner realms wisely, but also to protect you as you move deeper and deeper into them. Hallucinogenic substances are capable of catapulting you deep into inner spaces where powerful beings who guard life, death and the Abyss reside. Your mind has no interface with which to communicate properly with such beings; you are there without proper context, with no guardians, no guides, and often for no good reason. The chances that things can go badly wrong are huge indeed.

The more visionary magic you have done, the more chances there are for disaster to strike, usually by blowing a fuse in your mind. If you have spent a long time working in the inner worlds, your mind is already pliable. Adding a hallucinogenic chemical to the mix will push your mind deep into the inner worlds and beyond its boundary of capability.

So how come tribal magicians can work well and powerfully using these substances? Well, let's have a look from an outsider's point of view at how they operate.

When a tribal magician uses a visionary substance, whether it is to connect with beings, to heal, to attack, or to protect, they use the substance within a specific context. A tribal magician or shaman (or whatever you want to call them) works within a specific land radius, with particular spirits and beings of the land, with ancestors to which they are deeply connected, and with power spots that are close to the community that they serve. They are deeply tied to the land and its beings by nature of their blood line: generations of tribal magicians will have built up

## 1.11. Visionary and hallucinogenic drugs

a vocabulary and circle of spirit 'relatives,' along with a deep understanding of the spirit aspects of the visionary plants that are used and worked with.

All of this comes together when a tribal magician works, not only to ensure the success of the endeavour, but to also protect and guide the magician as he or she works. And the work is always done for specific reasons that involve other members of the tribe/community, or the tribal land. Such a tribal magician will also live in a very specific way, eat in a specific way and keep constant vigil over the land, its spirits and its people. This act of service is recognized by the local spirits, which is why they are willing to work closely with the magician.

This is not to say that what tribal magicians do is all sweetness and light—they will often think nothing of killing someone with magic if they are asked to and there is good reason. Tribal cultures tend not to be too infected with the New Age syndrome of thinking that everything is love and light.

The final, most important point is that tribal magicians tend to stay in realms close to our own. They operate within the inner landscape of the land and the threshold of death, and not much beyond that. There is no need to go further: with most of the jobs that tribal magicians do, these realms suffice.

Western visionary magicians however tend to delve far more deeply into the inner realms, passing across thresholds of time, walking deep into the inner desert, the Abyss, the stars, the angelic realm, the deep underworld, and so on. Once you have trained your mind to go to these places those pathways cannot be closed: any drug can place you anywhere within those realms without warning.

When Western-cultured magicians want to experiment with a tribal visionary substance, they do not think about setting, context, contact, or reason. They are generally in a place where they have little real understanding of the land and spirits around them. Most often the magician is not in direct contact with ancestors or with the spirits around them, and they are not on the land where the substance was grown. When a plant grows on the land, it does not grow in isolation: it is the sum total of all the other plants around it, the spirits around it, and the power of the land it sits upon.

The main reasons I have heard people give for taking such substances in a magical contact are things like 'exploring myself,' 'going on a vision quest,' or just general curiosity. If you are still 'exploring yourself' then you are not at a phase where deep

# 1. Knowing your body: part 1

visionary magic is appropriate. If you are 'going on a vision quest' then learn how to do it properly. There are no shortcuts and no excuses. If you want to experiment with your mind and with these substances then that is a personal choice; just don't dress it up as something that it is not.

If you are a ritual magician who does not use visionary magic and has no natural talent in that area then there is a reason to use such substances: if you need to make a direct contact with a specific being. To do this wisely and effectively there are some points to consider:

First you need to find a substance that your body can cope with and which is natural to the land on which you live. Learn as much as you can about the plant/substance, its effects on the body, its history, its mythology. The latter is the most important: the myths and legends surrounding the plant will give you clues as to which beings work with it or are accessed through it.

Then, go out onto the land where the plant grows, and sleep next to where it is growing. This is an important step: by sleeping alongside it, your deeper consciousness gets to know the spirit of the plant and the land beings around it—and they get to know you. It's about making friends with the beings that accompany the effects of the plant. This may offer you some protection when you come to work with the substance.

And most importantly of all, have a damn good reason for doing it, and by that I mean a magical reason, not a personal ego reason. That way, you are more likely to gain some form of protection when you try to contact the being you want to communicate or commune with—though such protection is not guaranteed.

If you simply decide you want to contact a demon to become a living god, use the LBRP to protect yourself and then digest a bag of mushrooms: the most that will happen is that a nearby parasite will be vastly entertained by your antics. It will have a great time telling you it is a demon and acting very 'demonic' for you while it snatches as much energy as it can from you.

Why does this happen? The inner worlds have many traps, boundaries, blocks and heavily-toothed guardians to stop idiots from gaining access to anything remotely powerful. Parasites are about the only beings likely to be connected to under such circumstances. The magician has 'an experience,' their imagination dresses the encounter in suitable 'demonic' dress, and suddenly they feel all-powerful and have become a 'god' in their own lunchtime. If they persist in this behaviour, then the draining-off of vital energy plus the damage inflicted on the brain by repeated use of such substances will result in a fragile, mentally ill egomaniac.

However, if you are a skilled, mature ritual magician with no visionary capacity whatsoever and it is imperative that you have direct contact with an angelic being, demonic being, dead person etc, then the use of such a substance under the right conditions and done only very occasionally should have no serious magical consequences —unless the substance is toxic and poisons you: then you are screwed. Use of these substances is always a second-best option, as the contact is usually fleeting, nonsensical and hard to use, hence the importance of developing proper visionary skills if you want solid, usable contact.

If you choose to use such substances for entertainment, then that is a different matter entirely and has nothing to do with magic. In my opinion, that is down to personal choice and personal responsibility.

## 1.12 Chemical shit-storms

Last on this list of how to blow up your mind and your body are the chemical shit-storms we surround ourselves with every day. A skilled magician uses many different senses of their body and mind in their magical process, and an important and often overlooked one is the sense of smell.

A magician's sense of smell is an invaluable tool with a number of important and hugely beneficial uses. The use of plant extracts and oils, for example, became an integral part of magical practice as soon as we discovered that we could use scent as a magical tool.

As a species, our sense of smell is vital not only for our health and well-being, but also for the way it operates as an early warning system. The detection and secretion of scents and smells plays a key part in our ability to communicate, to remember, to differentiate, to threaten, and so on. But in our rush to be 'civilized,' our societies have tried to manipulate that process through the use of chemical smells to mask, attract or otherwise communicate. Modern living has convinced us that we need to use a vast array of chemicals to survive our daily life. In an average day, a person will use chemical scents or scent maskers when they bathe, wash their hair, brush their teeth, wash their clothing, clean their house, use their makeup, perfumes, colognes, deodorants, drive their cars etc.

## 1. Knowing your body: part 1

Even women's sanitary products and simple pleasures like toilet rolls are heavily scented these days; it has become a very difficult endeavour to move away from the chemical shit-storm surrounding us.

The effect of this vast array of chemicals, besides their very obvious health issues, is to lock down two of our most vital magical tools: our sense of smell, and our own unique scent that communicates on our behalf.

It would be wrong to think that the complex action of scents works only in the physical realm: that is not true, and it is one of the many skills within magic that is being lost over the years. One's sense of smell can detect inner connections, beings, and dangers as effectively as it can outer connections and threats, and I know from real experience that this is the case.

Magically, the sense of smell is involved in identification on both sides: inner beings can recognize us through our scent, and we can identify various types of inner beings through theirs. When a magician is surrounded by chemical scents all the time, this subtle sense is severely altered and diminished; it can take some time to re-establish the sense and build upon it.

The scents we emit also carry information about our state of health. When we are sick, the subtle scents we emit undergo changes that can be noticed by inner beings (as well as animals), and when an inner contact that we work with detects this slight change in scent, they will often warn us. For us too, when our sense of smell is unhindered by chemicals and is consciously developed, we can detect certain types of disease in other people by their scent.

A classic example is feeling slightly hostile to someone for no good reason. Sometimes this can be caused by a subtle scent the person is emitting which signals that they are diseased with infection—or even that they have a spirit parasite infestation. In this case your hostility towards them is a part of your own body's defence system, and it is trying to ensure that you do not spend enough time around them to risk becoming infected with the same disease. Another curiosity I have discovered is that spirits, beings and ghosts that we work with or are close to can create scents as a form of identification: you learn to become aware of a presence around you by the smell that they emit. Sometimes it is their own scent (like recognizing the scent of a person who has died) and sometimes it is a 'signature' scent that the being has learned to present in order to connect with you. Other beings leave a scent trace as a part of their general

## 1.12. Chemical shit-storms

identity, the classic example (which has become a stereotype but is nonetheless true) being the smell of sulphur when an underworld or demonic being is present—unless of course your drains are blocked!

So how does a magician develop this sense, along with tending to their own scent? The first step is to rid your body and home of chemical shit-storms. We are told constantly through advertising that we need a vast array of chemicals in order to be presentable, clean and respectable. That is not true, and there are other less damaging ways to have a pleasant smelling house, car and body.

The ways that I have tackled this problem are as follows. For keeping a house generally clean, I use ordinary unperfumed soap in both bars and liquid form. I slowly discovered that despite what the advertisements said, the bathroom, kitchen and the rest of my home could be very well cleaned with soap and water, polished with beeswax, and nothing more. If I really have to use a product that is scented, I use it sparingly and rarely. I use un-perfumed shampoo and conditioners, and I do not use deodorants: essential oils are a great alternative if one is needed.

But houses, cars and bodies do get a bit stale sometimes, even in the best conditions. For this there are a number of more natural ways to keep things smelling nice that will not interfere too much with your inner connections. One is to use natural resins or oils in a tea light diffuser. (Incense mixes and sticks are not such a good idea, as many of them contain fixatives and chemical scents.) A pure resin like frankincense is the best form of air freshener, and as a bonus it will eject low-level parasites and other unhealthy beings from your home; a property it shares with many other pure resins.

Living like this can be tough. We are programmed these days to expect a house to be full of chemical scents, and any sort of smell like cooking, tobacco, or animals is badly frowned upon. And yet, when we work with inner beings, those are the smells they expect to find in a home; and the chemical smells we surround ourselves with today are often particularly abhorrent to ancestral contacts. For the car, just a few drops of essential oils on the dashboard will do the trick. Just choose carefully what you use: some can be soporific and that is not a good effect if you are driving! The same goes for scenting the body; if you are going out and want to smell lovely, a few drops of homemade essential oil scent is subtle, smells pleasant, does not knock out everyone around you, and does not interfere too much with

# 1. Knowing your body: part 1

magical connections. However, it is a good magical practice to learn to live without constantly covering yourself and your surroundings with added smells.

A good way to make your own magical scent is to start with a base of almond oil (not too much or it will dilute the scent) and add in two or three essential oils. Then drop a few grains of pure resin into the bottle and give it a shake. A nice mix is vetiver, frankincense and opopanax essential oils, with a few grains of frankincense dropped into the bottle.

When you are working magically, particularly in vision, it is best not to wear any oils at all, so that you learn to develop your sense of smell. It is very fashionable to wear oils while working magically, but this is a misunderstanding of how such scents should be used. Most oils and incense resins were used to clear a temple or church and only allow a specific frequency of being to enter the space. If you are working in several different realms, then resins and oils can sometimes hinder rather than help. Specific oils can attract certain types of beings and block others out, but first it is important to re-establish your own sense of smell.

Once you have finished working, it can be very useful to burn pure resins and to use oils to remove any magical residue from the space and from yourself. You can also use them just before any magical process to clear the space. If you are working as an exorcist in a space then it is a different matter altogether: using oils and resins while you work will be very helpful. Also, some deities like the smell of certain resins and oils, and if you are working directly with them an offering of the appropriate incense can earn you brownie points.

Overall it is wise as a magician to learn how to live more naturally, to develop a sensitivity to smells, and to take note of the reactions you have to certain people when you are not dowsed and surrounded by chemical scents. The longer you live in a clear environment, the more sensitive you will become to what is subtly happening around you. Slowly you will learn what type of magical actions need smells and which ones do not.

## 1.13 Summary

As a magician living in today's modern synthetic world, it can be very difficult to stay healthy, strong and sensitive without taking specific steps to alter your lifestyle. There is a great deal of pressure on people to conform to unhealthy modes of living and trying to stay healthy and centred in such an environment can be difficult. However, the payback is well worth the effort. It is also wise to ensure that you do not become obsessive or paranoid about everything around you: this requires common sense and understanding that we also have to live in this modern world. Pay attention to your body, educate yourself, and treat your body with the respect it deserves.

Chapter Two

# *Knowing your body: part 2*

## 2.1 Checks and balances: energy in, energy out

In today's world of specialization and compartmentalization of our knowledge base, it is very easy to become myopic in how we view the reality of magic in our lives. We often see magic as being something 'apart;' the mad relative hidden in the attic only to be visited on special occasions and certainly not included in our everyday lives. This is a big mistake, and one that is often made both in our magical practice and our understanding.

In this chapter we will look at how everyday energy dynamics are affected by the practice of magic, and how magic affects our day-to-day interactions with the world around us. This is of particular importance for visionary magicians and those who work deeply with inner powers and energies. Just as the world around us can affect how and why we do magic, magic can also affect our daily lives, the lives of those around us, and how we operate as humans.

Magic is fuelled by power, and as the decades of magical practice roll by our bodies shift and change how they process that power. On the good side this means that as we age, we become more sensitive and responsive to the inner powers and contacts that are all around us. On the bad side, we also become more vulnerable or reactive to those energies and powers as they express themselves in our everyday lives.

For the average person who is not naturally sensitive, these shifts of energy and power go undetected for the most part, as people tend to develop natural immunities against them from an early age. This is why it can often take a long time for a young magician to learn the foundations of visionary magic: first the filters and blocks that they built in their childhood have to be dissolved.

Every human is different, and how each human responds to energies depends on a complex mix of upbringing, natural senses, health, community, religion, and so forth. There is no

## 2. Knowing your body: part 2

hard-and-fast rule, but a fairly consistent one is this: if you live a life of visionary magic, it will alter how you react to and process energy and power. For some this change is dramatic, for others less so. But every magician needs to understand how these energies work, how we react to them, how they can affect us, and how we can learn to consciously navigate a healthier, safer path through life. So what energies and powers am I talking about?

When a lot of people live in close proximity to each other, certain energy dynamics build up. How that energy expresses itself depends on the culture of the people, the land mass they live on, their spiritual coherence, their general health and their overall behaviour.

For example, in a country or area where everyone is more or less involved in the same religious or spiritual practice, a particular energetic dynamic builds up where beings, spirits, ancestors, deities, temple patterns (and so on) all interact in a constant flow of communion and energy with the population. This gives that population a sort of 'herd immunity:' protection from a whole bag-load of parasites and other unhealthy low-level beings. It does not stop them all or stop them completely, but it makes for a less friendly environment for them.

You can test this for yourself. Once you have a good level of energetic sensitivity, go to a place, country, or land mass where everyone is under the umbrella of the same religion. Although the area will have all the same day-to-day issues that any human community has, one thing will become quickly apparent: a lack of 'dirtiness' that you detect in its people, its towns and its buildings. I am not talking about everyday outer dirt, but inner energetic dirt. Places that have a long-term or ancestral spiritual base tend to be magically cleaner simply because of how they operate from an inner point of view. And this tends to happen regardless of the religion's structure or its ethics: the spiritual base blocks out certain levels of beings and energies. (As an aside, such a place will also block out access to certain inner realms that are not conducive to the dominant religious structure: doing magic in such a place is like hacking through a jungle to try and find a path.)

When that spiritual base begins to break down or fragment, inner dirt builds up and more parasitical beings move in (India is a good example). Such a state of fragmentation is what most of us live with in this modern world. This is neither good nor bad, it just is what it is; but it is important as magicians to learn how to adjust and adapt to it. In an energetically dirty city, for example, it is easier to work magically because there are fewer blocks, but it is much harder (though not impossible) to stay clean and centred.

Such challenges are all part and parcel of being a magician and a human, and this is just one example of the wide variety of energetic impacts that we as magicians need to be aware of and adapt around. Let us now look at the aspects of daily living that can affect or impact a magician energetically, and the various ways we have of dealing with them.

## 2.2 Living or working in a city

Where you live has a strong influence on how you do magic. If you live in a city you will slowly develop a natural defence against the inner parasites, beings and spirits that live around such large clusters of people. This natural defence has to be taken into consideration when you embark on a path of visionary magic: not only will you have developed a 'thicker skin' that makes working in vision harder in the initial stages, but from the moment you begin working in vision, you will potentially become very visible to every energy-eating inner being for miles around.

This is why any magical system that works with inner vision (as opposed to psychological pathworking) has pretty tight visionary structures for magicians to work through in their first few years of training. These set paths 'tune out' your visibility: you take on a different frequency which in effect makes you vanish. If they cannot detect you, they cannot eat your energies! Many magicians use banishing rituals before they begin to work. But relying on this method, which was originally intended as a simple training exercise for beginners, will obviate the deeper and more powerful protection you can build up through good working practice.

As you work through the set structures, you will begin to make connections with inner contacts, and your interactions with them will bring about various shifts in your energy. Slowly these connections will begin to form new constant protections for you, which will make it a bit safer for you to do magical work in a crowded city.

What you will find, however, is that there are areas of the inner realms where it is unwise for you to work if you are operating in a city. Those areas will vary from person to person

## 2. Knowing your body: part 2

and city to city, so as a working magician it bodes well to pay attention to the after-effects of your work. If you find yourself becoming fatigued and slightly ill after visiting a certain realm, try visiting the same place while working out in nature, away from the city where you live. If working there does not present the same problems, then you will know that your city was causing the issue. It is all about experimenting: you gain your own knowledge and wisdom by paying attention and acting accordingly.

Cities can also fluctuate between healthy and dirty, depending on which inner tides are active, what is happening in the city at the time, and what is happening to the land on which it rests. If, for example, rivers are redirected, or springs are dammed up, or burial sites are disturbed, that can change the inner health of the city, sometimes temporarily, and sometimes forever.

As always, the key is awareness: if something shifts and your work is affected, take note of the shift and ask the following questions: has something happened to the land on which the city sits? Or is something powerful happening in the inner worlds, something which most likely has nothing to do with you but is affecting your work? Or is something happening within your body? One of the important skills to develop as a magician is identifying whether the source of a shift in power is within yourself, the inner worlds, or the land around you.

If you are getting drained of energy when you work in the city, then work outside the city, out on the land, and see if that makes a difference. If it does, then it is time to work with divination to see what is happening to the city itself.

The first thing I do when I visit a city that is very dirty (if I am going to be there often) is to 'open the void' in the city's centre. This is not a cure-all, but it does help to 'tune' the place from an inner perspective. In days past, most if not all cities and city-states had an active temple that allowed a two-way flow of power between the inner realms and the city. The level of 'tuning' the temple provided varied according to what type of temple it was, the deity worshipped there, and how clean or corrupt the priesthood was.

In more recent times in Western societies, churches, mosques, synagogues and monasteries provided this tuning by way of daily mass rituals, daily communal prayer, or the perpetual cycles of prayer that occur in monastic and convent communities. Such tuning does not directly affect how a city's

## 2.2. Living or working in a city

humans behave, but it does level the playing fields somewhat: fewer parasites and low-level inner beings hanging around means less chance that humans are going to be manipulated into behaviour that allows a parasite to feed. The 'tuning' also helps the city's energy to keep flowing so that it does not block up, stagnate and go rancid. Think of waterways and sewers: inner energy works along similar lines.

By opening the void and tuning it every time you go back to the city (or every day if you live there) you allow a small crack of the void to remain open and for energy to flow back and forth freely. You cannot singlehandedly 'fix' a city, but a daily or regular practice of void meditation, bringing the stillness into the space and holding it there, allows the tuning process to begin. Soon, other beings within the land and the inner worlds will pick up on what you are doing and assist you. They will not do it *for* you, as the city was built by humans and it is therefore up to humans to clean up the mess. But if you make the effort, then they will help.

If there is a church, temple, cathedral or other place of worship in or near the city centre, then visiting it regularly, sitting quietly and meditating on the void within the sacred space will help to amplify the effect. It does not matter what religion it is, only that it is a place that uses ritual and prayer in honour of and communion with Divinity.

The older it is the better, and this is because modern sacred buildings tend to be built using architecture that is fashionable rather than sacred and harmonic. If you want a really good example of bad modern architecture for a sacred space and you are in that part of the UK, visit Bristol's Catholic Cathedral at Clifton. If you want to know what trapped and dirty energy feels like, go and stand or sit in that place.

To feel a sacred, tuned space, go from Clifton Cathedral to the main Bristol Cathedral in the centre of town. It is like night and day. Bristol Cathedral is still properly maintained as a sacred space and it has beautiful and harmonic architecture. As a result the energy flows in and out unhindered. It is energetically and physically a very beautiful place to sit and meditate. Just be aware when you visit places like this that they are sacred spaces linked to a specific path to Divinity, and that path must be respected at all times while you are there.

# 2. Knowing your body: part 2

## 2.3 Empathy: other people and beings

Most magicians find that the longer they do visionary magic, the more empathic their body becomes. For some this is a natural dynamic, and for others it is something that develops over time. Some magicians never develop energetic empathy, so this will not necessarily be an issue for you. Our interactions with inner beings, realms and powers develop and refine over time. Just as a child has to learn how to interact socially, spot dangers and learn from good or bad experiences, so the magician also has to learn by trial and error how to conduct themselves in the realm of magic.

Just as in everyday life we constantly learn what to do and what not to do, so too will the magician constantly refine and adapt themselves to the flows of power to which magic exposes them. And just as in our outer lives, visionary magic has some basic rules which, when followed, help us to stay safe and healthy. But there are also more complex situations that the magician must address on a case-by-case basis, and a fair number of those involve our energetic reactions to other humans, inner beings, deities, and so forth. We learn by doing, by observing, and by interacting. Direct experience, and how we evolve from such experience, will determine how we develop our own safety mechanisms.

For those who do visionary magic, natural energetic empathy is both a blessing and a curse. The blessing is that you are far more able to reach deep into the inner worlds, to read the inner patterns hidden in the outer world, to detect beings in or around people and places, and to feel illness in others. The downside is that such empathy, if it is strong, can also be very draining and distressing. I am a natural empath, and I have worked with visionary magic for decades. This has strengthened my natural empathy in ways that have caused me numerous problems, but it has also made magical work a lot easier. So it is a double edged sword.

Whenever I go somewhere very crowded, like a cinema, an airport, or a busy part of the city, I can easily become exhausted and overwhelmed by the mix of energies, moods, physical conditions, ghosts, and spirit hangers-on that I encounter. Over the years I have developed a series of coping mechanisms for this, along with making some interesting discoveries about my inner senses. The methods I describe below may or may not work for you, but it will give you a starting-point for your own experimentation should you find that you have similar problems to mine.

## 2.4  Inner alarms

The more a magician interacts with inner beings and the inner worlds, the more their inner and outer senses fuse together to become more alert and responsive. When you work regularly and in some depth with visionary magic, your 'inner' sight strengthens and begins to operate in tandem with your everyday faculties, until eventually they fuse together and become indistinguishable.

Say for example that a beautiful person walks towards you, but they appear ugly, out of sorts, or simply 'wrong'. Others do not notice this and would question your observation: they see beauty where you see 'nasty'. What is happening is that you are seeing the inner and outer person at the same time. If their 'spirit' or energy is diseased, has parasites, is unbalanced, or is just plain nasty, your inner sight will pick up on that they will look 'wrong' to you.

Alternatively, you may simply feel hostile to them for no obvious reason. In my early days of visionary work, this was the strongest presentation I got of my inner alarms going off. Occasionally I would meet someone who, although they seemed nice, balanced etc, just did not feel 'right' to me. I would shrug off the feeling, not trusting it, and continue my interactions with them. Soon enough the odd feeling I had when I first met them would prove to have been right, and they would be revealed as unhealthy, aggressive or destructive in some way.

Like all senses, this one improves with practice, but it is also important to be able to filter it. Otherwise it is easy to become paranoid about everyone around you, and such paranoia left unchecked can be an early sign of mental illness. The line between the development of inner sight and of mental illness is a fine one, but it is nevertheless well defined.

A magician develops this inner sense in tandem with filters for it; a mentally-ill person does not. A normal person will not react to everyone around them; they will walk down a busy street barely noticing most of the people they pass. They will register only the ones who present a potential threat— A mentally-ill person will see potential threat in everyone .

A man following you on a dark night in a predatory fashion is going to put you on alert; someone simply walking past you

## 2. Knowing your body: part 2

is not. How do you learn to notice threats? By experience, social learning, maturation, and everyday living. Just as a child slowly learns from their parents, from being a part of society, from being taught and from direct experience, so the magician learns also.

Incidentally, the same mechanism that allows us to spot potential threats also allows us to also spot other magicians, priests/esses and mystics. Their inner light will be visible to you: they will shine, look familiar, and will most likely also recognize you.

## 2.5 Energetic boundaries

The other major skill a magician develops as a result of visionary magic is a more general energetic empathy, something which can become increasingly pronounced the more inner work the magician does. Their energetic boundaries become looser, which is part and parcel of deeper inner work.

A lot of ritual magic paths make use of daily banishing and protections. This leads to a sterile environment, and as a result the magician is not able to develop much in the way of magical contact skills. This in turn severely limits their capacity to work with any real level of power or to be sensitive to beings and contact.

This 'sterility' also creates another very serious problem: the magician never learns to differentiate between types of beings and powers, or how to adapt and behave around them. As a result, they see all inner beings other than the ones they are invoking as being the 'enemy' that is out to get them. Sadly this is becoming more and more a feature of modern magic. The rules of basic conduct in magic are more or less the same as in daily life: if you lock yourself away and never interact with people, you will never learn social skills, never learn how to tell the difference between good and bad people, and you will never fully be a part of the magical world.

The healthier way to develop as a magician is to slowly learn about the different types of energies, beings and powers, and how best to interact with them. Such learning is also important for everyday life when dealing with people: magic and daily life are part of one another they are not separate.

As you delve deeper into visionary magic, you will slowly develop a heightened level of sensitivity. You will notice that certain people drain you, and others energize you. You will

## 2.5. Energetic boundaries

start to pick up a great deal of information about someone by standing next to them, and you will find that you can accommodate them in your energy field if needed. This understanding of the plasticity of our energy fields is a key part of operating properly as a magician.

If someone is ill or parasited, they will drain off your energy. This can be halted in various ways, though it cannot always be stopped. If you are only going to be near them for a few minutes, then there is a simple visionary action that can stop it. First, focus on the void for stillness, and from there simply visualize a hardened barrier around you. As your skills in visionary magic develop, this action moves from being a psychological visualization to being an actual magical act. The focus on the void gives you access to power; visualizing a barrier puts that power to work.

If the person causing the energy drain is parasited or possessed by an unhealthy being living within or around them, then that being needs to know it is not going to get a dinner off of you. Mentally wafting sigils at it will work only in about 5% of instances: that language only works if the being understands it. I have found that the clearest and most effective deterrent is to make yourself as inedible and scary as possible.

To do this, after first focusing on the void, replace that focus with a drawing-up of power from the underworld through your feet. Once that power is in you, project a demonic mask-face filled with the power of the underworld. These actions do take visionary skill and magical knowledge, but they scare the shit out of low-level parasites and beings. The ability to focus instantly and then to project such a power image while appearing normal on the outside is a skill in itself. This is why basic visionary exercises done daily are crucial to a magician's development: You must be able to access your power and visionary skills at a moment's notice, anywhere and under any conditions.

This sort of technique will not work against a powerful nasty being hanging around or inside a human, but such an encounter is rare. I have found over the years that if for some reason I am not capable of handling such a being, I am steered away from the encounter by inner contacts. If I do come into contact with such an entity, which has happened to me more than once, then that is a signal that it needs to be dealt with.

The best method I have developed for such encounters is to instantly connect with the void and then call upon Divinity. I also silently call upon the angelic beings that operate on the

## 2. Knowing your body: part 2

threshold of the void. When I am filled with power, I breathe out with the intention of breathing the pure power of the Utterance into the space around me. I then direct the breath of Utterance at the being. I have found that by doing this, angelic beings will either pull the being into the void or 'wrap it' to disarm it. The act of using breath with Divine utterance is a passive one: I direct the power at the being in an act of mediation, acting as a bridge between the worlds. I do not direct what the power must do, only where it should go. The angelic beings will do the rest as is needed.

I never take beings out of people unless they ask. It is not the place of the magician to decide who has a relationship with what. I have two exceptions, though: if I find a being in one of my kids I dispatch it, or if a being in a person is driving them to kill, I dispatch it regardless. Such dispatching is not to be done lightly, and certainly not attempted if you do not know what you are doing. You could inadvertently end up as the new host, if you are not careful.

Bridging Divine utterance at the edge of the void will alert inner beings to the threat, and will trigger an inner response that will unfold over time. Your magical work is to bridge unconditionally the consciousness and power needed to put that being back where it belongs, which you do simply by opening the void and calling upon Divinity. By initiating that action, you become the catalyst for change.

There will be times in your life as a magician when you will become drained by being surrounded by lots of unhealthy people. It's important to avoid such situations if you can, as the inner beings who work with you will assume that since you know the risk and still choose to expose yourself, then that is your choice. They will not help you or protect you from your own stupidity.

If you have to put yourself in such a situation, it is time to engage the various skills you have learned to protect yourself, and the inner beings who work with you will also do their part to help. It's all about common sense. I have been terribly drained and made ill by sitting in a cinema, an unnecessary place I chose to go to even though I knew it would affect me. But when I have had to visit people in mental institutions, hospices, unhealthy towns and cities I have been perfectly fine because it was something I was doing in service; on those occasions the inner beings I work with helped, guided and protected me where necessary so that I could get on with the job at hand.

## 2.6 Talismans

Many people have asked me about using talismans to protect them from being drained by unhealthy beings. The issues around talismans are not straightforward and the use of them is something that, for a number of reasons, should not be done lightly.

If a person is a natural empath but has no wish to develop that skill or to delve into deep magical study, then using talismans will do them no harm and will protect them. Talismans used unwisely will arrest a person's inner development, but if they have no wish to develop further, then it is not an issue.

Similarly, talismans can be extremely useful if a person is at a vulnerable stage in their life (e.g. their childhood or teenage years), if they are suffering from a severe sickness, or if they are living in a dangerous situation like a war zone (in the outer world, not the inner). They are a short-term solution to a problem that eventually must be permanently addressed. When made properly, a good protection talisman will block out anything and everything: it is the equivalent of shrink-wrapping yourself. (By 'good protective talisman' I mean one that is connected to inner contacts and patterns, not some hokey confection sold by internet magicians.)

The downside of talismans is they tend to do a job that you are supposed to do for yourself. The majority of challenges we face are opportunities for us to grow stronger, to learn from, and become part of a larger team of inner beings and outer humans.

When you step onto the path of magic you immediately start to become more visible to inner beings. Some of those beings are helpful, and others are parasitical and unhealthy. Part of your development as a magician involves learning to tell the good beings from the bad ones, and developing the coping mechanisms, inner immune system, and inner social skills you will need to navigate the inner worlds. You may be more vulnerable without a talisman, but such vulnerability will teach you your weaknesses and limits. It is really important that you know your limits, so that you will know when you need to ask for help, and when to not overstretch yourself.

You can only learn those skills through trial and error and through direct experience. If you constantly festoon yourself with talismans and do banishing rituals on a daily basis you will never encounter enough beings to learn which of them are healthy and which are not. Just as a child who is never allowed

## 2. Knowing your body: part 2

to mix with other children never learns the skills they need to deal with them, so an overprotected magician never learns how to interact with the vast array of inner beings.

If you are naturally empathic it is even more important that you learn to cope with this faculty, and again the only way is through direct experience. This also helps to toughen up your 'inner skin' so that over time you learn how to filter out and rebuff intrusive low-level beings.

Even so, there are times when any magician becomes overwhelmed: on those occasions it may be better to use a talisman for a few days or weeks to gain some breathing space. The key is to use them rarely, and only when under serious threat or when a major timeout is needed.

### 2.7 Protecting and healing within your sphere

This is something that happens often as a magician whether you are doing it consciously or not. When you work in magic, particularly if you are walking a magical path of service, your energetic boundaries become loosened, so that your inner consciousness can flow back and forth in a more fluid way. This allows you to be fully alert in both the inner and outer worlds at the same time. It also enables you to interact more directly, from an inner point of view, with the land and with people around you: the land will recognize you as a magical worker, as will inner beings, ancestors, faery beings etc.

With the development of civilized living, and as a result of pressure from religions and cultural norms, we are expected to shun anything that cannot be touched, held, and quantified. Imagination is for children, inner senses are silly, and we are constantly told to be in the 'here and now.' That approach culminates in a locked-down adult who finds it very hard to be in touch with themselves, let alone any being or realm they cannot see.

Working magically in vision and practising meditation slowly peels back that hard layer and allows one's spirit to breathe and flow, which is more in line with its natural state: we become more attuned to everyone and everything around us. The more a magician works in vision, the more they are able consciously to affect their own boundary, and one of the benefits of this is the ability to take someone into your boundary of energy.

The magician learns to expand their energy field and to 'wrap it round' a person who is very vulnerable. This is not a skill exclusive to magicians: many natural empaths will nod at the concept of taking someone into your field to protect, heal or energetically feed them.

The question of learning such fluidity takes us back to a very basic working known as the 'vision of the void,' the key ingredient for so many magical actions. Once still, you expand your field of 'silence' beyond its normal boundary and envelop another living being with it. You will discover that other magical paths and mystical branches of religions have versions of this described in their mystical writings and meditational methods, if you look closely enough.

I use this method to help a child, a pregnant woman, a dying person, a sick animal etc. that is in need. Standing by them, sitting with them or holding them, expand your energy field beyond the both of you so that they are completely within your sphere. Then, deepen the void within you so that a deep stillness fills you and the person you are holding the space for. The first action brings the person into your frequency, which immediately protects them. The second opens the gates of the void so that power can flow back and forth. That is all you need do unless you have made the decision (and they have asked you) to give them direct healing or protection.

By holding them and opening the gates of the void, you act as an intermediary or door for any power, connection, or contact they need. This is an act of service. It is usually done consciously, but it can also happen unconsciously: you often do not realize it is happening until you suddenly feel the stillness all around you. You will be very tired afterwards because it is hard work, and you will most likely need to sleep.

## 2.8 Sex

Sex can be draining for a number of reasons besides bedroom gymnastics or prolonged marathon sessions. If one of the partners is ill or badly out of balance, then sex can cause a magician to become quite badly drained (the life is literally sucked out of them) and the out-of-balance partner feels great for a while. Another draining element can happen when parasites are involved, which is a lot more common than people realize, and is not always bad.

I will not go into much detail over this issue because I have written about this subject matter before (in Magical Knowledge II) and do not wish to repeat myself. Suffice it to say that if

## 2. Knowing your body: part 2

you find your energy becoming badly drained from sex, take a consecrated bath and ritually cleanse your home. If it is a parasite the draining will stop, but will very possibly creep back. If it is your partner, then no amount of cleaning will solve that one. They have to sort themselves out.

If you ritually cleanse yourself and then find that your sex drive drops quite a bit, then you know that a being was feeding on your sexual energy and was also boosting your sex drive so that it could get a more regular supper. Then you have to make a choice... live with the parasite and have a great sex drive but get drained, or have a more natural sex drive and not get drained. Such a decision is a personal choice: sometimes symbiotic relationships with such beings work in a healthy way and sometimes they do not—it's up to you to decide.

### 2.9 Raising kids

Having children is probably one of the most draining and rewarding experiences a person can have—and also the most frustrating, mind numbing and hilarious. Besides all the outer effort it takes to raise a child, it also takes a great deal of inner energy to raise one who is balanced and healthy. The ins and outs of the magical dynamics around children would make a book all of its own, and for this book the question of children is very much a side issue. Suffice it to say, if you are a magician and are planning to have children (and this particularly applies to the mother) then prepare for your inner resources to be stretched to the extreme.

Don't for a minute assume that you will be able to conduct a full magical life with a child around, particularly for their first 7 years. Raising a child is a major commitment from an inner point of view and you will find that your inner energies are almost completely devoted to protecting, nurturing, introducing, bridging, fighting off nasties etc, particularly when they hit their teen years. I was lucky, I had my kids young—I was twenty one when I had my first child, so by the time I was ready to begin deeper magical work, they were past the very vulnerable stage.

If, however, you find that your child suddenly and unusually drains you badly, and it has nothing to do with stress, arguments etc, then it is probably time to give them a ritual cleansing bath and do a proper cleansing of their bedroom. If that does not work, do a reading to determine if something dangerous is happening. The sudden draining could just be an unhealthy situation like parasites, or it could mean that your energy is being used to protect them or hold them back from a disaster, serious illness or potential accident.

This brings me to the other main reason for a drain of energy, which is working unconsciously to protect someone. This happens automatically with your children, but it can occur whenever you are closely connected to someone. If you have been working on someone who is very sick, then it is possible that that your deeper spirit will continue to work on them from a distance. Personally I have found that no matter how I try to cut connections under such circumstances, as soon as I fall asleep I go to the sick person, work on them some more, and then wake up exhausted. My inability to learn how to break connections has led me not to offer to heal (except for my own family/friends, and then only when it is absolutely necessary).

Getting drained is part and parcel of magical service, though not every magician will be called upon to work in protection and healing—it depends on who you are, where you are, and what you do. Some magicians are called into magical inner construction as service, others become guardians, or power weavers, or destroyers. There will always be, times when you will get drained, so learn how to deal with it. Just as working on a construction site at the age of forty five will knock the stuffing out of you, working hard in the inner worlds will tire you out at times.

## 2.10 Summary

There are times when the draining of energy is a strong warning that something is amiss. It tends to be my default major alarm signal: I suddenly deflate when something is wrong. An unhealthy landmass can drain you, an out-of-balance city or town can drain you, as can a sick person, a child, an unhealthy object brought into the house, deep magic, an incoming attack, a working tide going out—the list is endless. The key is to find out what is draining you and do something about it. The best way to identify the problem is through observation, and to identify the best solution using readings: look at your options and the situation that surrounds you.

Most of the time, particularly in the early stages of magical development (such as beginner or initiate) getting drained should not be much of a problem unless you are a strong

## 2. Knowing your body: part 2

empath. The deeper you go in to magical training the more of an issue it becomes, but it should still not become a major problem. If it does, then there are two possible explanations: either you are working unconsciously on a long-term project and your tide is waaaaay out (discussed in the next chapter), or you have overstretched yourself and are getting sick. Preventing that from happening, and dealing with it when it does happen, is essentially what this book is about.

Chapter Three

# *Energy and magic*

## 3.1 Paying the piper: the price of advanced magic

There is no such thing as a free ride, and this is particularly true for magicians. The majority of people who get involved with magic do so out of curiosity, or because they wish to connect deeper with the powers around them (mysticism), or because they wish to control their environment (results magic). All these paths have their own energy dynamics, issues, rewards and problems. Most magicians dabble in all types of magic at some point or other before they settle on what feels best for them and discover what they can cope with.

Part of the learning curve is to discover how the scales of magic work in your own life. Everyone will be different, but there are some inherent power dynamics that it pays to understand as early as possible. Learning by direct experience is always best. It is not so much the experience itself that teaches you, as how you respond to it that will polish or destroy you.

The information in this chapter it is not presented to you in order that you should totally avoid the situations discussed; rather it should give you a better understanding of the parameters involved so that you can make more informed decisions and react logically rather than emotively to some of the impacts that magic can have on your body.

I broached the subject of energy dynamics and magic in my book *Magic of the North Gate* and the following chapter expands on that information, looking in more detail at the energetic ups and downs that occur on the magical path. Forewarned is forearmed: if you have an idea of what could happen to you, then you can practice avoidance magic—otherwise known as the art of dodging bullets!

## 3. Energy and magic

### 3.2 Magic and energy

All magic uses energy of some kind, and the deeper or more powerful the magic, the more energy is used. Different kinds of magic use power/energy in different ways, and the form we practise will determine how that energy will interact with us. The whole picture can become very complex but the basic rule of thumb is this: externalized or ritual magic creates and mediates energetic patterns in this world, and then draws inner power to the pattern. Visionary magic or inner work creates patterns in the inner worlds, and then draws those inner patterns through us before externalizing them. Folk magic tends to nudge whatever is already present.

It is crucial to understand how and why these methods affect you in order to learn and grow as a magician. It is good to walk a path with your eyes open, and it is important to have a basic understanding of how to manage the downs as well as the ups of a magical life. Some energetic problems can be avoided with foresight; others cannot. For those that cannot be avoided, it is better to know how to mitigate their effects than to fall victim to them.

In this chapter we will look at the energetic dynamics of some of the various forms of visionary magic that most magicians use, so that we can see how they can potentially affect us.

### 3.3 Visionary and inner magic

Visionary magic takes many different forms and is done for a variety of reasons. How, why and where you act magically will determine what effect it will have on you. The sort of effect produced can vary enormously, from being filled with regeneration to being totally trashed, and some forms of visionary magic will have little or no effect on your body. It is all about level, context and content. In general, the deeper or more involved your visionary magic is, the more tired you will be afterwards—not because visionary magic is unhealthy, but because you will have worked hard and your body/mind/spirit is tired.

### 3.4 Bridging

This form of magic works with energies closer to the source of their inner pattern, and the magician interacts with powers,

## 3.4. Bridging

deities, inner constructs, contacts, beings and different realms through the use of visionary imagination. Because most of the action happens in the inner worlds, before it can have any effect in the outer world it must bridge through the magician, who acts as a mediator for the power. This simple act can knock the shit out of the strongest magicians, because the power has to pass through your body before it can go anywhere else.

The immediate effect of bridging is to be filled with power and to feel amazing: injuries vanish, your mind becomes crystal clear, your body glows with energy, and you appear youthful and strong. Once the power has passed through you and gone off to do whatever it was supposed to do, you will either return back to your creaky, grumpy old self, or if you are overworking you will dissolve into a puddle on the floor and feel like shit for days. Hopefully you soon recover, ready for the next bout of energy-boxing with the gods.

How much bridging affects a magician depends on what they are bridging and why. When it is an important job that you have been called or guided to do and you are only one of many other beings working on it, the effect is often minimal, even when the overall work is very powerful. Other times, if you are doing inner construction for example, or are working more or less alone, it can feel like you have been wrestling elephants once the power wears off. A magician who persistently overstretches themselves in the inner worlds or tries to grab power can literally end up destroying themselves.

Bridging works with a few different energy dynamics. One is where the power that you are bridging is far greater than your body was designed to hold. Even though you have no intention to hold it and are simply acting as a doorway for that power, it still fills every cell in your body before it passes onward and out into the world. This can be good or bad, depending on what power you are mediating, what that power does, and how healthy your body is at the time.

If you are working with an energy that heals, regenerates and balances, then its effect can be wonderful if you need it, and sometimes it is tempting to try and hold onto it briefly. If you do that but don't actually need any extra energy, it can sometimes 'overfill' the pot of your own energies and trigger an immune reaction which becomes inflammatory. Hence the wisdom of letting the power do its own thing and not interfering with its natural progress.

## 3. Energy and magic

If you are young and strong, then your body will adapt pretty well to the demands of bridging energy—unless you have already broken through into working with major powers. If that is the case, it is best to be proactive and learn to maintain your body and spirit so that you can withstand the heavy volume of work that awaits you without getting injured or sick. If you are older, it is wise to start keeping a close eye on your health, and be willing to adapt your working methods and actions if necessary.

When you work in the inner worlds, you stretch your spirit in ways that it is not used to: we do not grow up in societies where such inner actions are the norm and therefore practised from an early age. We are the equivalent of thirty-year-olds learning to walk for the first time after three decades of allowing our leg muscles to atrophy. It takes time to build the muscles up slowly, and if you overdo it you will get an injury.

If you are already working on bridging energies and beings, keep a close eye on your health and don't dismiss the subtle little whispers of discontent that a body tends to put out: pay attention, and act accordingly.

The subsequent chapters in this book look at a variety of symptomatic pictures and methods for maintaining and healing the body. No matter how good or strong different healing modalities are, each body works in its own way. Experimenting with different healing forms while tracking your health through readings will show you which forms work best for your body. Also bear in mind that any single healing modality will work for some things and not for others: you may find that you need to use a combination of them to support and heal your body after magical impact. Don't think in terms of constants and consistency, approach it more mutably and go with the flow.

### 3.5 Inner study

Working in vision to learn, observe and study has the least impact on the mind and body of all types of visionary magic. This is why it is very important to spend plenty of time as a relative beginner doing regular meditation and work with the void, and going into well-established and frequently-visited realms to learn. It is also very helpful to connect with a guide so that your mind and body become acquainted not only with the inner pathways, but also the energies of inner contacts.

## 3.5. Inner study

If you are still finding it a struggle to hold focus and quieten the mind, then you still need to be only practising and learning, not working or doing deep exploration. There is a phenomena to look for which will tell you that your body and mind is going through deep adjustments, and that is where the visionary process falls away and you find yourself deeply still to the point where you think you have fallen asleep or lost consciousness. But it is not the same as simply falling asleep: the deep shift closes off the consciousness as the power flows and yet you surface at the end of the vision.

This happens mostly when someone else is leading you in vision or you are using a recording: your mind is able to let go and the deeper spirit emerges to connect. But if you simply abandon focus on the vision and let go, the power shift does not happen. It is a paradox: by using focus to stay conscious, the consciousness gives up trying to interface with the imagination and the deeper consciousness connects directly with the power.

This is common in the early days of visionary work and it is a sign that you have made the crossing from the simple use of the imagination to an energetic interfacing with the inner worlds. It can still happen occasionally to an experienced magician, and it is often a sign either that the power you are connecting with is either unfamiliar to you, or that you have gone very deep into it.

This 'loss of consciousness' dynamic is very difficult to understand and work with if you are a lone magician, but it is not impossible. When you are working with a group and someone is leading the vision, the group energy upholds you as you work and whoever is leading the vision verbally acts as a beacon. If you do work in a group, it is wise afterwards for everyone to talk through what they saw and experienced. This helps to jog your memory, and even though you may feel like you had passed out during the vision, hearing other people talk it through brings back to you what you actually experienced: most of the time you did not fall asleep, you just went very deep. Whatever you experienced will come back to you when it is ready.

One of the key signatures that you all made it into the inner realms is that you all see the same things even though they are not mentioned by whoever is leading the group. With a psychological pathworking, which is not magical vision, you see what is described and have a few personal experiences as your

## 3. Energy and magic

imagination and personality use the pathworking to address personal issues.

With visionary magic, your imagination breaks through into the inner realms and you all have common experiences that are not described because you are seeing and interacting with what is actually in that realm. An interesting example of this is a group of magicians I know who are all lone practitioners and are scattered at various locations around the world. Recently they were individually drawn to work in the inner desert and all experienced an inner contact that I am aware of but have never described. Each one had a startling encounter with a powerful ancient inner contact that has a very specific description and each magician thought that their imagination had made it up. No, they had all tuned into a specific power as it flowed through the inner realms.

From a learning perspective this is why it is important not to second-guess, analyse or dismiss something you see in vision if it is outside your personal experience. For every contact, power and realm described in books, there are many more that are not spoken about; it is very important that you find them for yourself. You will get outside confirmation in one form or other, and you will also feel it in your body: a solid contact interacting with you changes you as you also change them—power/energy interactions between consciousnesses always bring about change.

But these learning interactions usually have only subtle effects and not the massive energetic impacts or rushes of power that work interactions can bring. For this reason (and also for obvious other reasons), if you are working as a magician in service in the inner worlds, it is good for your body and spirit to alternate work visits with learning visits, not only to give your body a rest but also to allow for a deepening of understanding both of mind and body.

In today's world of university education, the concept that you go to school for four years to get a degree and then you are an expert has had an effect on how we learn. The age that an undergraduate gets his or her degree tends also to be the age (your twenties) when you know it all and have a delicate ego. This is normal: we have all been there, and at the time most of us were so sick of being looked on as a student that we wanted to be taken seriously as an expert. I know I am being general here, but it is a reoccurring theme: once people have learned how to navigate the inner worlds, they want to get to work. Great. But it pays dividends in the long run also to keep learning. Keep working within the safer inner places like the Inner Library (the inner university for magicians and priests!) because you can never, ever, in a lifetime, learn all there is to be learned from such places.

The constant visiting of these places in order to study also helps the body to stabilize and learn. It is like doing your yoga before breakfast: you don't just do it to learn technique; you do it to maintain the body. Visiting the Inner Library and deep meditation in the void are both visionary versions of a 'morning yoga routine.' Use the simple visions as a part of your body and mind health routine. They will anchor you, teach you, and help your body regenerate.

## 3.6 Observing to bring change: magical exploration

This is a weird one and can have a really long pull upon your energy, or not at all. It is a dynamic that cannot be predicated because of its very nature. This power action is implemented in the inner desert (the landscape of the Tree of Life) where time, physical manifestation and death are woven together before spilling out into Malkuth (the world). Standing in the desert, particularly at the edge of the Abyss and observing the angelic power-patterns come together to create a filter (in Da'at) for the utterance of Divinity to pass through as it crosses the Abyss from Kether and begins its journey down the Tree (through the desert) is to witness the creation of life itself. By having a living human consciousness observing, the process is altered: we become a part of the process and that inclusion by observation brings change to the pattern.

Our energies interact with the pattern and that interaction can continue long after we have come out of vision and moved on with our lives. It does not happen every time, and there have been times I have observed and then felt no further connection to the process. Other times I have observed and subsequently felt the pull on my energies for weeks or months afterwards.

Through the act of observing we cease to be individual humans for a span of time and instead become timeless beings mediating change at the very edge of creation. If that change is going to manifest as something longstanding, our energies become entwined with the process and will continue to be so

## 3. Energy and magic

until it has reached its peak, at which stage it begins its slow descent into decay. The pattern of death begins at birth.

I discovered this action purely by accident and like everything I find in such a way, I work with it until I understand it a bit more. Over a few years of observing in this manner I have come to understand the process a bit better, though I do realize I am still only grasping one percent of it all. But I have noticed that when I observe a major coming-together of power, my energies can be tied up in it for quite some time. It is not all draining: some of the energy that comes from observing is inspiring and energizing—one cannot tell how it will affect anything until it does.

So if you are involved in this type of inner work, just bear in mind that your energy could be tied up for months or longer, though what you stand to learn far outweighs the potential disadvantages. I learned more about magic, power and mysticism from those observations than from any other magical practice. The only thing I would change in retrospect is that I would have timed my interactions better so that I was not partaking of such an act at a time when I needed full access to my energies for everyday life. Saying that, these powerful events have their own time and you fall across them when the time is right for all involved.

The first time I connected to this observation action, I was completely trashed afterwards. But as I lay on my bed staring at the ceiling, all my poor little mind could do was to say "wow... just...wow!" I learned more in twenty-four hours than I had in the previous ten years.

I have come back from such observations filled with power—and that power hung around for weeks. Like all exploration work, you have no real idea what is going to happen until you do it. It did however introduce me to the concept of power in observation, and when I finally learned how to magically observe an event taking place in the outer world, I realized that this brought through an interesting ingredient to the power mix. Not only can you change something simply by observing it, you can also become a passive mediator for power and consciousness to flow through. It is important not to try to direct or shape what flows through you; rather it is enough simply to be a bridge for whatever is coming through into the situation you are observing. You become the human version of the angelic filter that works at the edge of the Abyss, except you are working in Malkuth: we are substance-bound beings working through substance.

By passively observing and being willing to act as a filter in the physical world, you become a lower octave of the same process that is happening all the time in the inner desert. And it is important that you are physically there, looking with your own eyes: watching something on a screen does not work. (I know, I tried it.) It is the physical presence of the physical being that makes it work. I also found that I could only act as a filter in Malkuth after I had experienced the process in the inner desert in vision; the inner experience primed my spirit to be able to take up the role in the outer world. One startling difference is that while the physical observing triggered a lot of magical energy and 'did things,' it did not trash me the way the inner vision did.

Working in substance in a body on the physical plane may seem like the natural order of things, but I had to go through the inner experiences first to become aware of the act, to understand it energetically and to experience how it felt. Then I could consciously and actively participate in the process as a mediator/magician rather than being completely unaware of what was involved in.

## 3.7 Power weaving

Coming from a city of weavers, I found this particular form of visionary magic to be of great interest and took to it like a duck to water. The method of power weaving itself is described in my book *The Magic of the North Gate*, so I will not repeat it here.

Essentially, it is actively working with the weave of energy or power that brings fate, action and events into play. Whereas the angelic pattern filtering at the edge of the Abyss brings form into being (a person, a tree, a building, a genetic race), the weaving brings events and action into place.

When I wrote about power weaving a couple of years ago, I had fallen across it in its raw form and spent a few years essentially 'playing and tinkering' to find out how and why it works. But I had not been working with it long enough to know the prolonged effects it could have, how it affects the energy, the body etc. Now, a few years down the line, I have a bit more of an idea. But I suspect that my understanding of this work has not even begun to scratch the surface of its potential application and effects.

So far I have found that, although there seems to be no long-term energetic impact from this work, I get a 'twinge' when

### 3. Energy and magic

another being or magician connects into the power weave that I was working with, as though they nudge a little bell when they interact with the same weave. Working directly with the power weave is hard work, and afterwards I would feel like I had put in a full day's work at the mill. But that feeling quickly faded.

I find the twinges interesting, but am not sure how to interpret them. My guess is simply that once we weave into something energetically, we become a part of that weave and will therefore be aware when anyone else joins it.

It also reminds me of an experience I had many years ago when observing a weaving process between planetary beings. I attempted to hold one of the threads for a split second and suddenly all the beings were aware of me (uh-oh...). But I was too busy feeling like a building had just fallen on top of me to worry about lots of very tall pissed off dudes looking my way. I think I 'twanged' their weave, and I do not think they appreciated it.

If you work with power weaving in the inner worlds, keep notes on your reactions over months and beyond. Both you and everyone else could learn a lot from your experiments and experiences.

## 3.8 Energetic consequences of working with deities

The subtitle of this section sounds very doom and gloom, but it's not, although you do need to take certain things into consideration when working with deity powers. Much depends on how you work with them and what your intention is. If you are working with them as priestess or priest in a temple or worship scenario, then their impact or effect on you will manifest in a particular way. If you work with them as a magician, then you will experience a different set of effects. Both ways of working have their advantages and disadvantages.

As I have said before in my books, when you work with deities it is wise to tread carefully and pay close attention to what happens around you. More details on the general ins and outs of working with deities (how they are formed, etc.) can be found in my book *The Magic of the North Gate*.

It is also critical to differentiate between serving them as a priest or priestess and working with them as a magician. For this section I will discuss working with them as a magician and the

## 3.8. Energetic consequences of working with deities

effects, good and bad, that such work can have on your energy and body.

When you work with a known deity that has been worked with for a long time (i.e. hundreds or thousands of years) the pathways of power that they work through are well established and therefore can have predictable effects upon your body. The general rule of thumb is to check carefully what energies they work with and what they tend to do with them. Deities are not 'all-powerful all-knowing' beings: they tend to have specialities, limits and a particular focus. Just ensure that you work with one that has both positive and negative attributes, so that they are a balanced power.

Sekhmet, for example, has a balance of healing and destructive aspects, so her power, her knowledge and her applications can go either way. Her positive side also expresses through the goddess Hathor, who is part of the 'Sekhmet' power group. If you want healing, work with Hathor. If you want to know *how* to heal, then you need to learn both polarities of the power, which means working with Sekhmet.

If you work magically with such a power, it will fill you and work on you before it fully engages in magical tasks. So if you are generally healthy but for some reason your body/mind/spirit needs to go through a process of disease in order to mature or balance you, then working magically with such a deity as Sekhmet will trigger the necessary illness. This can be a bummer, but it is important to understand that it is also necessary, so work with it and help the process along.

Similarly, Sekhmet's destructive power can fill you with a sense of power that is beyond your natural capacity. It is important to understand that such power or energy is not your own: you are simply bridging it wherever it needs to go. If you cling on to it, you will spin out in a self-destructive cycle. The more deeply you work in visionary magic with deities, the more powerful your interactions with them become, and the more potential there is for it all to go horribly wrong.

On the positive side, if you work wisely with such power, it will trigger your body's own creation and destruction cycles, which will strengthen your overall healing capacity over time. If however you choose to work with a 'heated' power like Apollo (a solar power) and you have a fire personality or body type, then you are likely to trigger chronic inflammatory conditions unless you properly balance out the work with counter-powers.

## 3. Energy and magic

Magical work with deities tends not to be draining. If it is, then you are connecting not to a deity but to a parasitical being dressing up as one. But working with deities over a longer period of time can change how your body and immune system works. If you work with a particular power for extended periods, your body's structure, repair mechanisms and fuel begin to change to align more closely with the deity's power. Such changes are usually a good thing, but it is worth observing them closely so that you always know how your body is adjusting.

It is important to be aware of these changes because if you get ill and use alternative healing like homeopathy or acupuncture then it will not work in the usual way. Magic changes how the body responds to illness, and working directly with a deity will make that change far more pronounced and focused.

For example, if you caught influenza, your symptomatic picture would point to a specific set of remedies and treatment. But after a magician has worked in-depth for a while, the regular remedy will often stop working for them. Their body's parameters change, and its reactions cannot be relied on when choosing the right substance to treat the illness. The method of treatment has to be approached in a very different way, often in a more poetic way, by looking at the treatment in the context of the deity's powers and the work that has been recently undertaken with them.

This is where the tarot really comes into its own. You can use a specific spread to look at what is happening in the body and what effect a particular treatment would have. The choice of treatment and its potential action can also be tracked through tarot, and in the process you are often shown very interesting insights into how a substance works and how it relates to your magical activities.

So if you are working in-depth magically for a period of time with an ancient Titan or an ancestral sleeper, do not be surprised if your thyroid starts to run a bit on the slow side!

### 3.9 Conditional magic and body effects

Conditional magic is the use of magic for a specific result, and it is usually undertaken for the magician's benefit or by the magician on behalf of someone else. Conditional magic works very well, but like all forms of magic it has its price, and if you choose to use conditional magic then it is wise to know what that price can potentially be. (In this instance I am discussing

## 3.9. Conditional magic and body effects

only the energetic and bodily implications of using conditional magic; its deeper, spiritual implications are a different matter altogether.)

A lot of conditional magic relies on the cooperation, sometimes forced, of a being or beings. If a being is forced to undertake a specific task, then the use of that force requires energy, which is usually drawn from the magician's own reserves. Sometimes that can be an issue; other times the magician rebounds quickly.

The long-term energetic implications of forcing a being's cooperation can sometimes weigh the scales of balance against the magician, as it can divert much-needed energy not only from the resources used for their body's upkeep, but also energy from their fate/life path. The magician often does not notice this until much later in their life: a dangerous situation occurs and the resources that should have been there for them to be able to safely navigate it have been used up and are no longer available. So before you decide to force a being's cooperation for conditional magic, first use divination to look at the long-term implications for you of such an action. Sometimes the price is worth paying, and sometimes it is not.

Another form of conditional magic uses the assistance of beings that freely cooperate with you. Although this is more ethical than forcing a being to act on your behalf, it can have even more damaging consequences if it is not approached knowledgeably. Many of the beings and spirits that will offer you help with conditional magic are parasitical in nature and will work for you very effectively, but for an energetic price. If the bargain and boundaries are not struck properly, then those beings will take their wages by way of your life force, leaving you to slowly weaken and sicken. Or the energy can be taken from your 'fate pot,' a deeper store of energy that surfaces during potential disasters to help you navigate, survive and learn.

If such energy has been drained from you (and this can happen without your knowledge if you do not know how to keep an eye on it) then your potential for surviving or avoiding fateful disasters or illness is severely reduced. There is no such thing as a free ride, and if you decide to use conditional magic then it is imperative that you state what price you are willing to pay: 'I will give you *this* and no more if you are willing to act on my behalf'. If the being you are working with is a land being, an ancestor etc, they tend to honour such deals (they will work for precious objects, power substances etc.). But parasitical beings

### 3. Energy and magic

tend not to be so honourable, and they will take what they want regardless of your boundaries.

When a magician gets into long-term parasitical relationships, it slowly begins to show and what is happening becomes obvious to anyone with inner sight. The magician will slowly begin to look grubby and unhealthy, their mental stability will begin to fragment, and repeated chaotic and destructive incidents or behaviour will become a major feature of their lives. When a person displays these symptoms it does not always mean that they are becoming a victim of their own magical practice: such patterns can emerge for a variety of reasons. But when a magician does conditional magic and is not very careful, such a pattern will very likely emerge.

What type of being is willing to work with you depends on what you are trying to achieve. Not all conditional magic is 'bad,' it is simply a dynamic that can quickly become destructive for your body and your general life if you do not tread carefully. So if you are using conditional magic, ensure you know exactly what you are working with, establish tight boundaries and exchanges, and watch your physical and mental health very closely.

## 3.10  Long-term projects

Some magical work, either service or inner construction (of a lodge or temple for example), can have longer-term energetic effects on the magician, often in ways that are unpredictable or unexpected.

When we are asked by inner contacts, deities or ancestors to undertake a task, we are often not aware of the ripples into the future that such action can cause. Similarly what can seem a short-term action or one-off working in service can in truth take years to unfold, and as that unfolding occurs, so our body's energy is woven into that action until its completion.

I did not realize this for many years, and would happily take on major short-term workings in service which at the time did not seem too strenuous at all. (In fact, some powerful actions often feel like not a lot is happening while you are working, so it can be difficult to ascertain just how much power is flowing through an action until it is finished.)

Here is an example. A few years back I was asked to go physically to an ancient temple and do a magical action in service. I did as I was asked and it did not physically feel too demanding as I was working: the contact was very strong, the action went smoothly, and it all made sense. An hour after the ritual finished, the two magicians who were guarding me as I worked suddenly became quite ill, but they recovered after a couple of days and that was that, or so we thought. But no, magic is never that easy.

Things started to change in the manifest world around the temple. Some of the changes were quite dramatic, and each of them had a direct effect on the three of us who had been involved in the ritual. We would suddenly become exhausted for no reason, which each of us separately put down to our health or our workload. It was only when we got together and compared notes that we realized our bouts of exhaustion were happening to all three of us at the same time—and in relation to outer world events around the temple where we had worked.

This is still an ongoing situation. Just when we think it is settling down, it all kicks off again and the three of us lay around drooling for days. Would I change anything in retrospect? No, I do not think I would, except this time I would do readings to look at the long-term effect on all of us before I initiated any action, so that any side-effects can be planned for.

It is not that the work we did at the temple has made us ill, rather that we are still 'working' at an energetic level at key times in the process. So be careful what you sign up for! Just be aware that often magical work has a longer unfolding cycle than we realize; if you have undertaken magical work that is operating directly upon something that is manifesting major change, then your energies are going to go up and down with the tide of power as it flows in and out of the situation, place or construct.

## 3.11   Ritualizing the action

One way to diminish the impact of powerful inner work is to make sure that if you working in depth with a large amount of power, either alone or in a group, then give your inner work an externalized ritual form to ground it and help bring it out. Do not try to do a lot of advanced power work only in vision. You are the first bridge into substance for the power; ensure that it passes through you and into a ritual pattern which will help it to take form and stabilize before it goes out into the world to do whatever it is going to do. The ritual acts as a substation for the power: any backwash hits the substation —the ritual—before it hits you. The ritual acts as a power buffer.

## 3. Energy and magic

It is these buffers that are handed down though the generations, and when they fall into the hands of young magicians they think they have found a powerful ritual that will do X. Sadly (or thankfully) for them, all they have is the external substation of the power, not the power button itself.

### 3.12 Retirement: knowing when to back out

There will come a time in a visionary magician's life when the body or spirit is no longer able to provide the necessary resources to continue visionary work. This is usually a time of transition, where the magician's work shifts and changes into a different form.

The magic may become more exteriorized through ritual, or it may become a natural flow whereby the magician no longer actively engages in 'magic' but magical power flows through their everyday life in a constant act of 'magical living.'

Working in visionary magic puts a tremendous strain on the physical and spiritual body, and the more adventurous or exploratory the work, the shorter the magician's working life will be. Usually magicians quickly learn that when using deep visionary magic, the actual act of vision does not need to be done regularly: less becomes more in terms of work. It should be just one element of magical practice, not the whole thing.

When it is time to stop, you will know. The idea of going into the inner worlds will fill your body with a sense of dread, and your instincts will tell you that it is time to retire. If you go with the flow, you will experience a shift in your own power over months or a couple of years. The power of the visions will be all around you in everyday life: everything you do will be an echo of the decades of visionary work that you have undertaken. The magic comes to you, finally. A simple ritual act will be filled instantly with power and contact without any conscious need to 'plug in' or work from an inner aspect.

Slowly the magician is taken from being a person who conducts magical acts to being a person who is magical. You turn up somewhere, and change happens. You step onto land you have not visited before and the landscape, creatures and weather react. You have externalized that 'change through observation' dynamic so that you slowly become aware that it is happening all the time, all around you.

This can be a very special time, a beautiful time, when you are able to take a breath, step back, and watch the awesome show that is creation.

## 3.13 Summary

Before you can do anything about a problem, you need to know what the problem is. Always keep a working diary so that you can track not only the unfolding of the magical work that you do, but also its effects on your body and mind. To do deeper magic and expect it not to have any physical impact is as much folly as thinking you could hike to the South Pole or build a house without any physical impact. Bruises are going to happen.

The key is to know what is happening and why. Are you tired because you have worked hard? Are you tired because the work is still going on? Did you get injured, or are you still carrying something around and are not aware of it? Have you been impacted, attacked, or has a being ridden back with you? Have you successfully completed something but taken a knock and your body is out of balance?

Once you have pinpointed the possible cause of the issue and identified the symptoms, it is time to find the appropriate cure or care. It is also wise to know how to avoid such impacts in the future.

Chapter Four

# Symptoms, reasons and power dynamics

## 4.1 The reactor reaching critical mass

Now that you have a general background of how advanced magic can affect your body, let's look in depth at magical actions and the more specific types of physical backlashes that you may encounter.

Often but not always, the types of physical or mental effects you can suffer as a result of deeper magic work relates directly to the type of being or power you are working with: certain parts of the body are more vulnerable to specific types of power and contact. It is always good to remember that these mental and physical effects are not visited upon you intentionally by beings; it is only a side-effect of their power.

Working in depth in magic is akin to working with volatile and dangerous substances, or to practising an extreme sport: there will be accidents and injuries from time to time but if you work intelligently, with safeguards, these impacts can be kept to a minimum. And if you do take a hit of power that affects you badly, then you need to know how to ameliorate its effects and how to help your body recover.

Similarly, it is important to be able to differentiate between a 'good' magical impact and a 'bad' one. A good impact is where you have successfully achieved a magical action and the body effects are transitory; you have worked hard and you really feel it afterwards. A bad impact is where you have overstepped a boundary, clashed with a being, or reached too far into a power that is not meant to be accessed by a human. Hacking into uncharted territory will often bring a mix of good and bad effects: it takes a lot of energetic effort to break new ground, and it is very likely that you will encounter a being that is hostile or at least incompatible with human contact.

Let's look at the various types of impact, their causes, and how they affect the body and mind. Bear in mind that this is not an exhaustive list, but it will give you a background to work from.

## 4. Symptoms, reasons and power dynamics

Everything listed here is something I have either experienced myself or treated other magicians for.

## 4.2 Magical impacts

Magical impacts are just that: you do magic, you get impacted, and your body suffers the consequence. A direct hit is not something a beginner would normally experience simply because there are too many filters across the inner worlds and deeper powers: someone in the early years of magic will not be able to get anywhere deep enough (usually) to injure themselves.

For more advanced magicians though, it is a different story. These types of impacts tend not to hit ritual magicians who do not use vision, as they are caused by direct inner contact. Exteriorized magic without use of inner contact or vision by its very nature filters and blocks such impacts because ritual without inner work blocks and filters deep contact. But if you are a visionary magician or a ritual magician who also works in vision, then your chances for getting injured begin to climb as you push deeper into the inner worlds. Such injuries will not happen regularly. They are usually the result of very deep work that is often experimental or 'archaeological' in nature: breaking into old disused patterns, forbidden thresholds etc. So do not think that you will be injured every five minutes, but it is very likely to happen at some point.

Why does it happen? Magical impact is usually the result of interactions with a power that is beyond your body's capacity to cope with. Just as we humans interact on a subtle pheromone level with each other, so in the inner worlds, beings (including humans) interact subtly at an energetic level. If you are communing with a being that is vast, then the chances are its power will prove too much for your body to cope with.

A similar effect can happen when you are dealing with pure power: when you work magically with power it always flows through and around you. If the power is of a high level, your body will freak out or get 'burned' by it. The other main cause of injury or impact in the inner worlds is moving too quickly: falling through the worlds and literally landing with a bump, or being grabbed by a hostile being.

Let's have a look at some examples of what has happened to magicians (and to myself) when they have been impacted. This allows you to put the information into a context and to see how it unfolds.

## 4.3 Examples of impacts

Many years ago, when I was even more stupid than I am now, I was an avid explorer of the inner worlds. I loved pushing boundaries to the extreme, as I always wanted to know what was beyond the horizon. One such round of work took me deep into the Underworld, in search of the ancient power of the planet itself. I wanted to know what made it tick; the nature of the consciousness of the Earth's core. I did manage to make it quite far down (though not as far as I wanted to go) and I had a strange interaction with what I presumed was the consciousness of the threshold of the Earth's mantle. When I came out of vision, I burned. I was so hot my skin was tingling as though I had sat too close to a fire. I lay down for a while to let it pass—but it didn't.

I had to get my act together, as otherwise I was going to be late picking my kids up from school. My kids asked me why I was so red, and when I got home and looked in the mirror, I saw that my face was sunburned—in the middle of winter. I put some aloe vera on my skin before going to bed and thought nothing more of it. I had experienced something similar a few years before, when I was working with an underworld deck for the first time. Then, the effect had quickly passed.

That evening I became sick. I developed a fever and I burned all through the night. The following morning I did a health reading. The picture showed I had something akin to radiation poisoning. So I started taking Kelp tablets for iodine, and over a few days the fever finally settled down. This was not a major impact, but it permanently changed how my body reacted to power. The immune response it triggered has become a learned behaviour for my body. Ever since that time, if I come into contact with magic that springs from that Underworld source, I burn, go red, and then have a few days of inflammatory reactions throughout my body.

My big all time idiot impact that changed my health permanently was the bright idea I had to mediate the Goddess Kali into substance. I was young and had absolutely no idea what the hell I was doing. I took four days to do the work, two of which I worked around the clock. To cut a long story short, I ended up with scarlet fever and permanent physical damage, as well as a longstanding pattern of strep infections that were really tough to fight at times.

What caused the illness was my lack of knowledge coupled with my natural ability to tap into power. I had already worked

## 4. Symptoms, reasons and power dynamics

with Kali for a long time, and bridging her into substance (i.e. a physical form like a deity statue or painting) seemed to me a natural progression of my work with her.

Because I did not know what I was doing, I did all of the bridging myself. I did not know at that time how to filter power through other beings, how to work in a line properly with inner priesthoods, or how to prepare my body properly. I just did it.

My body was not ready to have such a destructive force flowing through it, and the power came through unfiltered and hit every little imbalance in my body : it magnified them many times over.

It was a harsh lesson and it took many years to rebalance my body from that impact, but in doing so I learned a great deal about bridging power, what it does, how it works, and so on. After that, whenever I took on a large project, I would first look carefully (through divination) at all the parameters. I would prepare my body properly, ensure that I was working with a team of inner beings, and I would spread the process out over months.

The culmination of that learning process was understanding how structure worked, how inner powers flow from one world to another, how teams worked, and how to anchor the work properly so that my body did not take the full impact. The result of that learning is presented in my book The Work of the Hierophant, which goes into depth about bridging and building at an advanced level.

I have also come out of visions with black eyes, a dislocated shoulder, and a torn ligament. This sounds pretty extreme and the product of an overactive imagination, but it is not. It does not happen that often, but the impact of contact with a powerful being like an angel can certainly knock the body about a bit. It tends to be a direct injury that heals naturally. Think of Jacob wrestling with the angels: he had contact with angelic beings and he got an injury. It is exactly the same dynamic with visionary contact. Usually when I get injured it is because I am either fighting something, carrying something very heavy, or I am doing something stupid. Most of the time after a vision, I feel only the strain of making the contact..

Another interesting example is an impact sustained from an encounter with pure power. This happened to a magician friend of mine that I have a lot of respect for. He is a natural magician and also a very well trained one. But like all of us he makes mistakes, because that is what we do and how we learn.

## 4.3. Examples of impacts

This magician had been working in depth in the inner desert with the land powers around him and with threshold contacts. The work had been slowly building over months, and the power was becoming more and more intense. He was reaching for the formless power, and wanted to bridge it unconditionally from inner to outer. He worked in his temple, opened the gates, and mediated raw power.

What came through was so strong it triggered alarm reactions in various magicians around the world: the power was too raw, too unfiltered, and was full of destructive potential. He quickly closed the contact down and closed the gates, but by then he had already sustained an injury: the power had flowed into him and through him, damaging his brain as it passed through.

Luckily the immediate side-effects were strong enough to drive him to seek help: he began to wake with crushing headaches and a horrible feeling that slowly got worse. He was manifesting a brain injury. Even though nothing had physically touched his body, the impact of power was great enough to elicit a reaction in his body, which reacted as though it had sustained a head injury. If that impact had been left untreated, it would have snowballed into a permanent physical head injury. He was sensible enough to contact another magician who immediately prescribed a series of strong herbal treatments for a head injury (*hypericum perforatum*). With the use of the herbal treatment the headaches and horrible feeling eased and finally stopped.

Although it was a frightening situation and very painful for him, he learned a great deal about bridging power and how to filter it. It does seem to be a reoccurring theme that we magicians sometimes have to learn the hard way. In this case, it was his first real experience with a major power impact, and in many ways it was very necessary: you can read about it as much as you like, but until you experience a direct hit, the reality of the power levels that magicians sometimes work with are often not understood, accepted or even believed. In every serious magician's life there will be an impact somewhere. The key is to know how to deal with it, learn from it, and adjust accordingly—hence this book.

The most usual form of impact after a work that magicians experience has no lasting effects, and consists of disorientation, followed by vomiting. It only tends to happen after a group working, and therefore the levels of energy being worked with are high.

I do not know the biological mechanisms of why these injuries and reactions happen; only that they do, and that

## 4. Symptoms, reasons and power dynamics

maintaining the body carefully will help to lessen many such reactions.

## 4.4 Magical imbalances

This is an area of magic and bodily health that truly fascinates me: the imbalances within the hormone system that can occur as a direct result of magic. The body's hormonal response to power really demonstrates how magic works *through* the body, how the body responds to magic, and how inner power is processed by an outer container (the body).

Understanding the very basics of how the endocrine system functions will help the magician to watch their body carefully and respond to any disturbance brought about by magic. The endocrine system is usually the first thing to react when the power levels worked with are too high, or the work has been done too quickly for the body to assimilate it.

Magicians often presume that a bodily reaction is the result of an attack or injury, when in fact it is simply the body reacting to a power overload. This is why it is important to understand the different ways that the body can react to magic, so that the right steps can be taken to treat it and protect its integrity.

When there is a problem, the first glands to trigger alarms are the adrenals, the thyroid, and (as a result of the thyroid reaction) the ovaries in women, which will affect their menstrual cycle. Let's have a look at each gland's reactions to magical impacts, and the cascade of symptoms that can result.

## 4.5 Adrenals

The adrenal glands sit over the kidneys and are our body's early warning and reaction system for danger: they provide us with the cascade of hormones necessary in order for us to deal with a dangerous situation. When we are under threat, the adrenals swing into action and give us quick access to energy, keep us alert, and reduce any inflammation in the body.

When a magician bumps up against a powerful being or a dangerously large amount of power, their adrenals swing into action and provide their body with the resources it needs for 'fight or flight'. When the adrenals are healthy and not overused, an adrenal response during a magical act will feel like being filled with energy—something that also happens as a result of tapping into flows of power.

## 4.5. Adrenals

When the adrenals activate, we become hyper-alert, our heart rate increases, and we feel very aware of any potential danger. This sort of reaction is not a problem unless the magician works regularly with powerful forces and deep contacts: the adrenals will become fatigued by the constant triggering which in turn can weaken them.

One way to avoid such burnout is by regularly working with the meditation of the void, or with similar meditations where the magician learns to still the body and mind, silence the emergency reactions, and approach power with calm stillness. It is not something that can be achieved easily and it takes practice, hence the need for regular or daily meditation, particularly at the neophyte and initiate levels of work. The initial reaction of the adrenals still happens, but it is muted and quickly dissolved.

If deep work is not approached with stillness then problems will eventually start to surface. Adrenal reactions are also heavily tied to emotional reactions, so if a magician approaches deep and powerful work with an emotional agenda, then detachment and stillness is impossible, as the engine is primed for reaction. Powerful magical work with an emotional agenda, for example to 'fight for the goodies' or 'slay the baddies,' puts the magician into a 'war' situation which puts the adrenals into full swing.

If on the other hand the magician approaches powerful work with the intent simply to do a job that is necessary, or to be a part of a working team with inner beings, then the lack of emotional attachment makes stillness easier to achieve. Anyone would find being in the midst of a riot or battle extremely stressful, regardless of their reasons for being there. Very few people would find cleaning the toilets or the kitchen stressful. How you approach the work will define what frequency of power you find yourself interacting with.

Let's look at a hypothetical example. Let's imagine that a lot of power was building up in the inner worlds, and that the emerging power was destructive. As humans, our understanding of time and of the long-term evolution of a change is very limited, so we cannot tell whether in this case the destructive power is necessary, good, or just plain nasty. But inner contacts that work with a magician—let's call him Fred, tell him that on this occasion, the inner worlds need a human's help. So Fred decides to answer the call and go work in the inner worlds. He builds the ritual structure for the power to flow through which is necessary in order to work deeply, and then he goes into vision. He goes into the inner worlds with an attitude of saving

## 4. Symptoms, reasons and power dynamics

the world from 'nasties' or from destruction—in other words, primed for battle. This approach immediately defines Fred as 'conditional,' that is, he is working towards an outcome that he wishes to define even though he does not fully understand what is happening.

As a result, many of the very powerful beings (usually angels) who work with this sort of massive energetic weaving to bring about change cannot use him as he would become a 'spanner in the works.' And as a result, Fred cannot penetrate the angelic frequency, so he cannot see them.

All that is visible to Fred are the beings mediating the destruction rather than the beings weaving the future pattern, and the former are often demonic, conditional beings. As far as Fred can tell, he has stepped into an inner realm full of powerful demonic beings bent on mediating destruction from the inner to the outer.

That would certainly set anyone's adrenals going. And because of Fred's limited perspective, it would be impossible for him to ascertain who should be worked with or what should be done. His situation becomes akin to a toddler on a battlefield.

The alternative scenario would be Fred answering the call and setting up a ritual pattern to support the work, but this time going into *stillness* before going into vision. By working without emotion or agenda, Fred appears at a frequency of the inner worlds where he sees only what he needs to see. Because he is still, unemotional and without agenda, the angelic beings can work with him without risking a human going feral on them.

Fred appears in the inner worlds and immediately feels all of the power flowing around the destructive pattern. But this time an angelic being appears, hands him a thread, and asks him to take it out to the outer world and anchor it in the land.

Fred does as he is asked; job done. He has experienced no encounters with demonic beings, no fear of the destruction, no battle-ready adrenals—but a powerful act has occurred. A being (human) of physical substance but with the ability to cross into the inner worlds took a thread of power from a destructive pattern, mediated it from the inner worlds to the outer world, and anchored it in substance: as a result the power has become connected to the vessel which is Malkuth. Since the power was mediated by angelic consciousness, whatever expresses itself as a result of that initial magical action is guaranteed to be necessary.

By performing that action unconditionally and in service, Fred has actively engaged in the Divine cycle of creation and destruction. Active engagement without the need to control triggers the octave of Divinity within humanity. That has wide-reaching implications not only for personal evolution, but also for the collective evolution of humanity.

Back to the adrenals. Had Fred acted conditionally, he would certainly have triggered his adrenals in a big way, and by exposing himself to such dangerous and conditional forces, the adrenal reaction would most likely have continued on for some time after the work had finished. His body and mind would have stayed hyper vigilant for days or even weeks, and for good cause: magic does not stop the minute you blow out the candle, finish the ritual or come out of vision—that is the just the beginning. The magician's spirit and mind (in dreams) would have continued to bump up against those powerful beings over a prolonged period of time. Within weeks, the adrenals would have started to show signs of fatigue.

If Fred acted unconditionally, he would still have had an initial adrenal reaction, but it would have been much less intense and would have faded quickly as the work was conducted blind: the mind could not perceive the threat and therefore did not react as much. The adrenals would have reacted to the initial rise in power, but when no discernible threat was identified would have settled back down. The unconditional Fred is more likely to have simply suffered a muscle strain from carrying the thread out into the manifest world.

So how do you know if your adrenals are overworked or getting badly affected? The symptoms of adrenal fatigue caused by magic are the same as those caused by 'normal' adrenal circumstances. First comes the hyper vigilance, headaches and sugar cravings. Then comes the energy crash, craving salt, being tired all the time, a drop in blood pressure, and the inability to cope with any stress. Later, the ankles start to swell from fluid retention, sleep patterns are affected, and allergies become far more pronounced.

These symptoms can also surface if you work unconditionally or blind for too long with large amounts of power. If your adrenals begin to show signs that they are struggling, it is time to back off the inner work and let them heal. If the health of the adrenals falters as a result of magic, then it is important not only to rest them, but to treat them.

If you are working at depth in magic there will be times when you will not be able to avoid triggering an adrenal reaction, but you can still reduce the severity of its effect. It is imperative for

## 4. Symptoms, reasons and power dynamics

an adept to know the signs of adrenal trigger (flight or fight) and adrenal fatigue, and to develop a sensible working practice to minimize any long-term effects.

## 4.6 Thyroid

The thyroid gland is another major player in the body, and among many other things is basically your engine's governor. Magic can directly affect the thyroid, though for some reason this more often affects women than men. The thyroid and its hormones control your metabolism, growth, body temperature, muscle strength, and appetite, along with supporting the health of your heart, brain, kidneys, and reproductive system. It is a pivotal gland that needs protecting from any kind of impact.

Magical impact of the thyroid is often insidious and builds up gradually, though I have come across acute impact in a couple of priestesses. Most often the first sign of trouble is a disruption of the menstrual cycle: the power of the inner contact or realm unintentionally 'tweaks' the thyroid which responds with a rapid shift in hormone output, which in turn triggers menstrual bleeding: the woman starts to bleed in time with the magical working rather than her usual cycle. Fascinatingly, the bleeding is often not a result of the magic itself, but happens in preparation for an encounter with power: the priestess begins to bleed on the morning of the magical work, not after it.

This phenomenon is connected with the 'tides of power' that flow out and in with magical work. The power of a major working begins to build the moment the decision is made to do the work, and the magician's body responds to that build-up. I always began menstruating just before a major working or a coming-together of magicians to work, and I understood from very early on that magically-triggered menstruation was connected with the tides of power. But it was years before I linked it to a thyroid impact—I can be a bit dense sometimes.

A thyroid reaction in the form of menstrual dysfunction is a very common magical reaction for many female magicians and priestesses, and seems to be of no major consequence so long as it does not happen on a regular basis or trigger endometriosis, which is a possibility. An easy way to support the thyroid in this type of reaction is to take kelp (iodine) for a few days before a major working and for a week afterwards. This way, the thyroid is supported and does not go into decline from the disruption. Just don't overdo the kelp: too much iodine is as bad as not

## 4.6. Thyroid

having enough (and if you live in the USA you will probably not need it or only need one kelp tablet before working, as iodine is added into food salt by law)

In fact, for any magical action that could possibly cause thyroid impact (if you know you are going to be working with deep or heavy powers, for example), take kelp just before, during and after the work. You cannot stop the impact that power has on the thyroid, but you can do a lot to lessen it. In these situations, look on exposure to powerful magic much as you would exposure to radiation: you often cannot get out of its way, but you can lessen its impact by how you attend to your body.

So what happens if the thyroid is not attended to and is regularly hammered by large amounts of magical power? The gland can go in one of two directions when it is impacted. In general, but not always, magical impact will cause a woman's thyroid to slow down, and a man's to speed up. That is a sweeping generalization: don't forget there are always awkward folks who have to be different... So learn the signs, and watch your body when you do heavy work. Don't assume that because you have testicles, your thyroid will not go on strike.

When the thyroid has been knocked out of balance and has slowed down, the person begins to feel tired all the time, feels cold and hungry, and nothing will warm them up or satisfy their appetite. Their hair begins to look dull and brittle, their nails break, and the distribution of fat in their body begins to shift. Sometimes people get an ache in their lower throat (over their thyroid), and their voice may become deeper.

If you have been doing powerful rounds of work and one day you realize that your body is grinding to a halt, then it is possible that your thyroid is not a happy bunny. That is the time to take action, and also to use divination to look at your thyroid's health, as well as the general health of your endocrine system.

Sometimes a slowing thyroid does not indicate a problem with the thyroid itself, but is caused by a magical impact in the pituitary or hypothalamus. The point of impact can sometimes be ascertained through divination (discussed in later chapters), and if it originates outside of the thyroid, you will have to treat the impact-point as well as the thyroid itself.

But the first thing to do in response to a slowing thyroid is to take kelp and to stay on it until your body feels better, however long that takes. Once you are on the kelp, then it is important to work out which healing modality would work best to get the endocrine system functioning again, and to ensure that you

## 4. Symptoms, reasons and power dynamics

attend to it. Also be aware that you can take too much kelp: follow the dosage advice on the bottle.

The thyroid has to be very out of balance before it shows in blood tests, but if you have a severe enough reaction it is wise to see a doctor, have blood tests, and take any necessary treatments. If your thyroid impact is severe, it is very important to have it attended to medically, even if you do not like allopathic medicine. You will not be able to do *anything* without a properly functioning thyroid.

Most of the time such an extreme reaction is rare, and if you use your common sense, spot the early signs, and treat it accordingly, it will never become a major issue. Such careful attention to the body used to be a major survival mechanism, and in pre-industrial times the magician (along with everyone else) would pay far more attention to their body's signs of distress, however subtle they may be. With today's super-baseball-bat steroids, antibiotics, antivirals, vaccines etc. we have become complacent and tend to ignore or not even notice the body's distress signals. We think that taking a pill will make things better—a sweet honeymoon of medical science that is slowly coming to an end in many areas of medicine. Learn to respect and care for your body!

With men, the thyroid is more often poked in the direction of hyperactivity, and although this is not a common reaction that men have to magic, it can happen in sensitive people. If, after working powerful magic, any man finds that they have difficulty sleeping, develop a fast heart rate, become anxious, and start to lose weight—and these symptoms continue for days and beyond, then the time has come to see a doctor. Do not try and treat a hyperactive thyroid yourself: it is a major health threat and can quickly get out of hand. Such hyperthyroidism in men as a direct result of magic is very rare to see, but I have come across it. As with all things magical, learning comes from first-hand experience and observation and not just studying: without paying attention, there is no progression.

### 4.7 Gland summary

The more I have observed physical reactions in magicians, and studied those reactions through readings, observations etc, the more I have the sneaking suspicion that the hypothalamic-pituitary-adrenal axis is thrown into slight disorder through severe magical impact. When the HPA axis is disturbed, it can cause a cascade effect through the endocrine system, affecting the above-mentioned glands along with disturbing a woman's menstrual cycle and generally causing fatigue, issues with body temperature, metabolism, and so forth.

Similar disturbances can be observed in people with post-traumatic stress disorder, and my guess is that prolonged and profound magical impact, or a serious long-term magical attack, can trigger a similar response to PTSD in the body. I am not a doctor and there are obviously no medical studies that have looked at the physical effects of magical impact, but after years of observation I have seen the similarities too often to come to any other conclusion.

## 4.8 Magical catalysts

A magical catalyst is where a magical action triggers a healing crisis within the body. Sometimes this is simply a side-effect of magical work being done, and sometimes it is triggered intentionally by an inner being that sees an imbalance within you and initiates an action that will trigger a healing response.

Often when the body is triggered in this way, it is not simply a passive healing crisis whereby an immune response is triggered, the magician rides out the response, and is all healed at the end. Life is never quite that easy. A magical catalyst will bring unresolved issues with your body or mind into sharp focus, and will awaken or strengthen grumbling problems so that they become more visible. Expect any issues with your body or mind that you have been ignoring, or were not aware of, to be brought right out and shoved in your face.

Examples of this are a grumbling sore throat or a skin issue that suddenly explodes and becomes painfully acute after doing magic. Or a minor allergy to something unhealthy suddenly becomes a major issue. Whatever is out of balance will be magnified: any unhealthy foods or substances that you ingest will start causing major immune reactions.

Essentially, if you are not properly paying attention to your body and it is beginning to struggle, then the issue will be magnified until you 'get it'. This only tends to occur when the problem could eventually lead you down a very bad road: an inner contact or being happens to spot it and they decide to take action.

It is all about personal decision and choice. The balance of self-responsibility versus help from the inner worlds is always

## 4. Symptoms, reasons and power dynamics

a fine set of scales. Inner contacts can show you things, guide you, act as a catalyst for you and so on, but how you choose to respond to their help is up to you, and your decision will dictate your future wellbeing.

So if, for example, a being triggers a response in your body and your immune system subsequently swings into action, you have two choices. You can either deal with it properly, which entails finding out exactly what is wrong, what caused it, and how best to treat it to restore balance; or you can ignore it or suppress it with drugs. The choice is yours.

Usually when an inner being acts as a catalyst for some bodily issue, this indicates that now is a prime time to tackle it. If you do take action, you will tend to find that help is guided towards you, and healers are put in your path who can help you. It can often take time and patience to heal imbalances that have been festering for a while, but such diligence pays off in the long term.

The best way I have found to differentiate between an impact and a catalyst situation is through divination. The deck you use is irrelevant, so long as you are familiar with it. What is important is to use a good layout and to phrase your questions carefully. (See Chapter Five: Tarot Diagnostics.)

### 4.9   Beings and the disturbance of the mind

This is one of the greatest dangers of powerful magic—though thankfully, depending upon how good your magical methods are, it is also a relatively rare problem. I mention it here only because it does sometimes happen and a magician needs to know its signs and symptoms, and what to do if it happens to someone they work with or they recognize it within themselves. Please also bear in mind that some of the symptoms of this problem can also manifest in more common and much less dangerous conditions. Here are some examples.

### 4.10   Intrusion

This rare occurrence is very similar to a real possession (which is also very rare). If a being has half-pushed its way into you and is trying to push you out entirely—and any type of being can do this—it is important to be aware of it. You will feel 'half in' or 'half out' of your body, and you will be aware of a foreign being's presence within you. This is different to mental illness, and none of other symptoms that indicate psychosis will be present. If you

## 4.10. Intrusion

catch the intrusion at this stage, it is relatively easy to get rid of it. Music is an excellent tool to ascertain what type of being that you are dealing with: certain pitches or sounds will suddenly become unbearable to you. When you find that sound, play it around you before you go into vision to tackle the intruder: this will loosen the hold the being has over you.

When you are ready, go first in vision into the void and be still. You will be able to observe the being better while you are in the void, and you will be able to ascertain without emotion why it is there and how it arrived. From that point, step out into the vision of the desert and walk to the edge of the Abyss. This is as far as one can get to the foot of Divinity when you are in such a situation. Call upon the Keeper of the Abyss to take the being from your sphere, and then call upon the angelic beings that work in that space to repair your boundary so that it cannot get straight back in again. Once you have done that vision, take a ritual salt bath, and then create a talisman to beef up your boundaries for a week or two. (See appendix for ritual bath and talisman methods.)

It is very important to understand how your body acquired a lodger, and how to prevent it from getting another one in the future. At this level of magic there is no step-by-step instruction: these sorts of events form part of your learning process, and it is important for you to learn how to get rid of unwelcome guests for yourself, how to repair yourself afterwards, and how to be more vigilant in the future.

As I said earlier, this happens very rarely, and usually not at all if you have a good magical working practice. Doing a banishing before a working or festooning yourself with protection will not work—if you are so locked-down, you cannot work at the power levels where such an incident could happen anyway.

What can cause such an event is working at a high power level without engaging the inner structures that come with their own inbuilt protection. Going off the beaten track into a high level of power can leave a magician vulnerable to an intrusion unless they are connecting with Divinity and working with the appropriate angelic structures for that realm. The other thing that can make a magician vulnerable to such an intrusion is intent: if you go deep into the inner realms with a self-centred agenda, then the powers that work with creation and destruction will simply ignore you: your wants and needs are totally irrelevant in the deeper realms.

## 4. Symptoms, reasons and power dynamics

If the being manages to get right into your body and push you out, then your everyday consciousness will not be focused anymore and it will be up to your deeper spirit to fight its way back. The one thing that can save a magician in such a terrible situation is a good understanding of the Qliphoth and its relationship with Divinity. Your body is a Qliphoth—that is to say, a vessel or container—that houses a spark of Divinity, a pattern that was established at your conception. A deep awareness of your relationship with Divinity will act as a safety mechanism, and one that will allow your spirit to re-establish its Divine right to inhabit that shell until your appointed time of death.

Such deep awareness is not a conscious thought that can be engaged like a weapon; rather it is a profound relationship between yourself, your body, and Divinity; a relationship that is established on a daily basis through your recognition of Divinity within you and all around you. That relationship is built up through daily simple meditation, and an awareness of Divinity within all substance.

This is why there are no shortcuts in magic: the simple tasks, meditations, rituals and visions that are used to slowly build a foundation for the magician to stand upon cannot be avoided or circumvented. If you try to do without them, and you still manage to reach deeply into the inner worlds and commune with power, then your lack of foundation could prove your downfall.

Such a foundation does not just come from joining a lodge or learning lessons; it comes from daily simple disciplines, the willingness to take your time to learn skills carefully, and a constant awareness of just how unimportant you really are.

Thankfully most magicians learn well, work carefully, and as a result do not encounter an intrusion; or they are stupid and because of that stupidity, never gain access to the realms of power where an intrusion could happen. But there are always exceptions, however rare, and one must always be prepared.

If you come across a magician who has been pushed out of his body and another being has moved into it, it is pointless to try to fix the situation yourself: the spirit of the magician must engage the rebalancing dynamic for themselves at a very deep level. All you can do is to go into vision and talk to their deeper spirit. You will usually find them at the side of the river of death. They will appear in the same way as many coma patients do: still attached to life via a cord, but unable or unwilling either to move forwards into death or back into life. When you find them, remind them of the Divine allocation of their shell (their body), and tell them that they must call upon the powers of Divinity to guide them back into it. After that, it is up to them. Magic is, above all other things, a school of soul-learning. That learning can be embraced and engaged, or it can be ignored and avoided.

## 4.11  Beings meet viruses in your body

This is a weird one, and it is also a fascinating one. It took me a few years to realize this was happening, but once my suspicions were aroused, I started to watch closer, to track the situations through readings, and to treat people accordingly.

What seems to happen is that certain types of inner-world beings also have a presence in our realm, and they have the ability to communicate with and enliven viruses lying dormant within the body. The being triggers the virus, which then activates, and the person gets sick. But as a result of the being's influence the virus acts in strange ways: the symptomatic picture is different, as though the virus had learned different ways to operate within the body, which in turn affects the body in very out-of-character ways.

This seems especially true of the herpes family of viruses. This is very interesting to me, as in biological terms a virus is not technically a life form as we understand it, unlike a bacterium or a fungus. In such situations it seems that either the virus 'changes its programming' in response to the inner being, or the inner being learns how to manipulate the virus to affect the body for its own ends. I'm not sure which it is, but the change in symptoms is very definite, and the virus itself tends to have a much more aggressive impact on the body.

When I first spotted this phenomenon in magicians, I would furiously treat them using my normal homeopathic and herbal methods, but the virus seemed far more resistant to my treatments than usual. When I looked in vision at the infected body, I saw a fascinating interplay between the virus (which appears as the viral structure trying to integrate itself with the nervous system) and another being. It took a while after spotting that (I'm a bit slow at times) to understand that I should try to deal with the being, not the virus, to see if that would settle things down.

So I started to experiment in different ways to eradicate the being, first through ritual bathing and cleaning, which didn't

## 4. Symptoms, reasons and power dynamics

work, and then by having the magician ingest consecrated fluid. When that didn't work either, I went into the body in vision and manually hauled the being out of the magician's body. That did work. After I had removed the being and safely disposed of it, I started to treat the magician in the normal way. Now the treatment worked to a point, but either the pattern of the magician's physical relationship with the virus had changed, or how the virus operated within the body had been permanently changed. So I had to adapt how I chose remedies and treatments. Thinking sideways solved the problem.

Through the years I was confronted with several similar situations in sick magicians, and over time I learned that the best results came from a mixture of visionary work firstly to remove the being, and then more visionary work to communicate with the body. The communication with the body using vision was needed in order to inform the various organs and central nervous system that the virus it thought it was fighting had adapted rapidly, and was now possibly a composite of virus and inner being. After that, I would use homeopathic and herbal treatment.

This combination shifted the body's response mechanism to the virus, and helped it adapt to living alongside the virus without having an immune reaction. This seems to work better than fighting the virus directly and beating it into submission.

When I have used this method, it has usually been to help magicians suffering either from one of the various forms of herpes (it is a pretty large family of viruses) or HIV. But it is also worth considering if you are infected with a strain of hepatitis. In fact, if you live with any dormant virus that could pose a health risk, be aware that certain beings could trigger it back into action, and if that happens you will need to help your immune system to deal with it. It should also go without saying that if you have a potentially serious virus in your system, and it activates, your first action should be to go to a doctor. Magical healing work should always be conducted alongside allopathic medicine when treating moderate to serious illnesses.

I do not know if this relationship with viruses is intentional on the parts of these sorts of beings, or if it is just a matter of 'wrong place wrong time.' When a being has attached itself or has moved into the body (not a possession, but more of an 'infection'), it is important to strip that being out before you do anything else. Often these beings are similar to parasites: they are small, low-level entities and seem to get themselves

## 4.11. Beings meet viruses in your body

into other living beings so that they can set up home. They do not necessarily affect the magician's mind or consciousness, but they can affect bodily functions.

Another instance where this can happen, and where it is definitely not deliberate on the being's part, is where the power/energy communion between the magician and the being accidentally activates the virus. This can happen with powerful angelic contact: the power surge that can happen from working with angelic beings in vision can sometimes trigger latent viruses within the body, subsequently swinging them into action.

In these cases, I think that either the immune system gets geared up by the inrush of power and goes off looking for a fight, or the virus is reawakened so that the magician can learn how to work with it. Some of these illnesses cannot be cured, but how the body lives with the virus can be changed: it is often the body's immune reaction to the virus that causes the problem, and so the way forward may be to shift how the body responds, rather than fight the virus.?

Most of the time, good working practice usually prevents these sorts of problems, but they can occasionally happen to anyone working in any depth in the inner worlds. Think of it in terms of catching a cold from going into the city and being around a lot of people. Basic hygiene and common sense can usually keep you healthy, but there are still going to be times when you catch something. It is back to the old mantra of pay attention, and act accordingly.

Chapter Five

# Tarot as a healing tool: layouts

## 5.1 Peering through the looking glass

The use of divination as a healing aid is as old as healing itself. The divination itself would often take many forms, and spirits would be consulted in the ancient process of 'diagnosing' and healing a person. Today most magicians use tarot only as a divination tool, but it can also be used as a vocabulary to bridge communication between a spirit and the magician, or it can be used to find things, assess things, and choose the appropriate direction. One of the hallmarks of a magician is the skill of being able to see what is coming, assess its impact, and decide what option to take. That skill can be focused down to a fine art in the use of tarot as a spiritual diagnostic tool. I first began using tarot in such a way in my early twenties, when I discovered that I could use readings to see what was going on inside a body. I had read tarot for nearly eight years by that time, but up to that point I had only used it vaguely and without any real focus (and I was only a child). Necessity forced my hand in my early twenties: I had a very sick baby, and the doctors did not know what was wrong with her (it turned out eventually that she was allergic to milk).

For the first couple of years, I was not very successful in my experiments with diagnostic tarot: my limited knowledge and my inability to think clearly certainly sabotaged me. I did not give up, though, and my perseverance paid off. And once my babies grew up and I was no longer sleep deprived, I had a bit more time to experiment. It was then that I learned how to create filters in my mind so that I got the information that I needed without lots of information that I didn't. And that is a major key to using tarot.

Many tarot courses these days use a lot of psychology, a lot of terminology from ritual magic, and a lot of psychological translation. Such courses proliferate not because such an approach works; rather it is taught that way because it pads

## 5. Tarot as a healing tool: layouts

out a curriculum that in turn makes money. These days it has become the official way to learn tarot, and yet learning in such a style can really limit a reader. I learned the old-fashioned way: at the kitchen table when I was still a kid—and the rest was lots of practice.

I use the Rider-Waite deck throughout these tarot chapters so that you can easily get a copy of the deck and work with it as you learn these layouts and interpretations, and because its images are a common language that everyone can relate to.

## 5.2 Points to think about

Before you dive into body readings, there are some things that you need to think about. When you look at the cards, remember that you are reading for a body and mind, and nothing more. Focus your mind upon the question at hand with the intent that each card laid down relates directly to something that is going on inside the body.

Do not be tempted to fall into psychological interpretations, spiritual interpretations, or life event patterns. When you want to know what is going on inside a body, using the right layout and the right reading approach (along with having a clear question) is the way to get the answer that you need.

Simplify your card interpretations down to bodily functions and magical energies. It can really help to choose single key words for each card, and put a label on each card with the keyword upon it. I have put a selection of key words for the deck in the appendix.

For example, in a health reading, the eight of fire/wands means a lot of fire power, which can indicate inflammation or a fever, or if it appears in a threshold position for the spirit, a magical fire attack. It does not mean that 'the person is experiencing an up-draft of energy that is going to take them on a journey where they experience new things.' Get my drift?

Remember that the idea of doing a reading to look at the health/condition of a body is no substitute for going to a doctor. I do both: if I am ill, I will go and see my family doctor, but I will also track my health through readings and use various alternative remedies. I let my doctor know what herbs I am taking, and working together like this covers all bases.

Finally, be aware of the layout you are going to use before you use it, so that it becomes second nature to your brain. If you want communication to filter through the pattern, it helps to know the pattern. As you shuffle the cards, be aware of the layout in your mind, or map it out on a piece of cloth so that you can look at it as you shuffle and then lay the cards down upon it. Once we have looked at the layouts, we will go on to look at the processes of shuffling, interpretation, and extending the reading to get more detail.

## 5.3 Layouts

Some of the layouts presented here are also to be found in the Magical Knowledge series or The Exorcist's Handbook, and some are not. I just thought it better to put them all together here so that if you are reading this and you do not have a copy of The Magical Knowledge Series, you do not have to buy it to continue this chapter!

The specific health layout in this chapter will tell you what is going on within the body, and that is usually the best place to start. From there, you will need other layouts to ask the specific questions that come up as a result of the first reading—to obtain clarification, for example, or to find the source of the disturbances. Sometimes the health layout on its own will give you the answer that you need. Remember that this is about a body, so your questions and interpretations need to reflect that perspective.

When you ask a question, be very specific. If you ask 'show me the health of the person X', you may only get a snapshot of their health on that day. If you ask a question like, 'show me the health of the person X for the next two weeks,' then you will get a better idea of what is going on for them. If it shows a disastrous pattern, then repeat the reading in order to look at the person's health over six months. If the disaster vanishes from the reading, then you know that the health crisis will be short-lived (perhaps a bout of flu, or food poisoning) and the longer-term health is fine.

## 5.4 The health layout

The health layout (fig. 5.1) is just that: it is a layout that gives you a snapshot of what is happening in the different areas of the body, and how they are affecting each other. This is an excellent place to start when looking at a magical impact that is physically manifesting, or an illness that is rooted in magic.

## 5. Tarot as a healing tool: layouts

This layout looks at the interaction of three forms of energy: emotion, inner energy coming from outside the body, and the energy the body derives from whatever it ingests. These three dynamics are inextricably linked, and the layout shows how those interactions affect the body's various functions.

**The first position** shows what magic, power, and energetic influence is coming from the inner worlds in order to manifest in the body. This is where any magic that could affect the body will show up; for example an inner contact, current inner work, or a magical attack. It is also the position where you will be able to see any future patterns of fate or action that have not yet fully begun to manifest. If the only negative influence in the reading occupies this position, then the destructive pattern is still forming and can be obviated or avoided, as it has not yet reached the individual's inner landscape.

**The second position** shows any inner influence that has already penetrated a person's sphere/has entered their inner landscape, and is now present in the immediate future pattern of the person. Something that turns up here is already having an energetic influence on how a body is operating, but it has not yet fully manifested as a full-blown condition.

It is in this position that we see the consciousnesses of viruses and bacteria, along with beings, magical attacks, impacts etc. Whatever occupies this position is already affecting the person's energetic body, and if left unchecked will descend into their physical body and cause symptoms.

Learning how to discern the meaning of the card in this position will really help you to understand what type of magical impact or injury you are suffering from. If something major shows in this position, do a follow-up reading using the inner landscape or desert layout to gain more detail.

**The third position** tells us what is physically going regarding the health of the head. That includes the brain, sinuses, lymph glands, endocrine glands in the brain[1], ears, nose, eyes, and the throat including the Thyroid gland—basically everything above the base of the neck.

---

[1]The hypothalamus, pineal, and pituitary glands.

5.4. The health layout

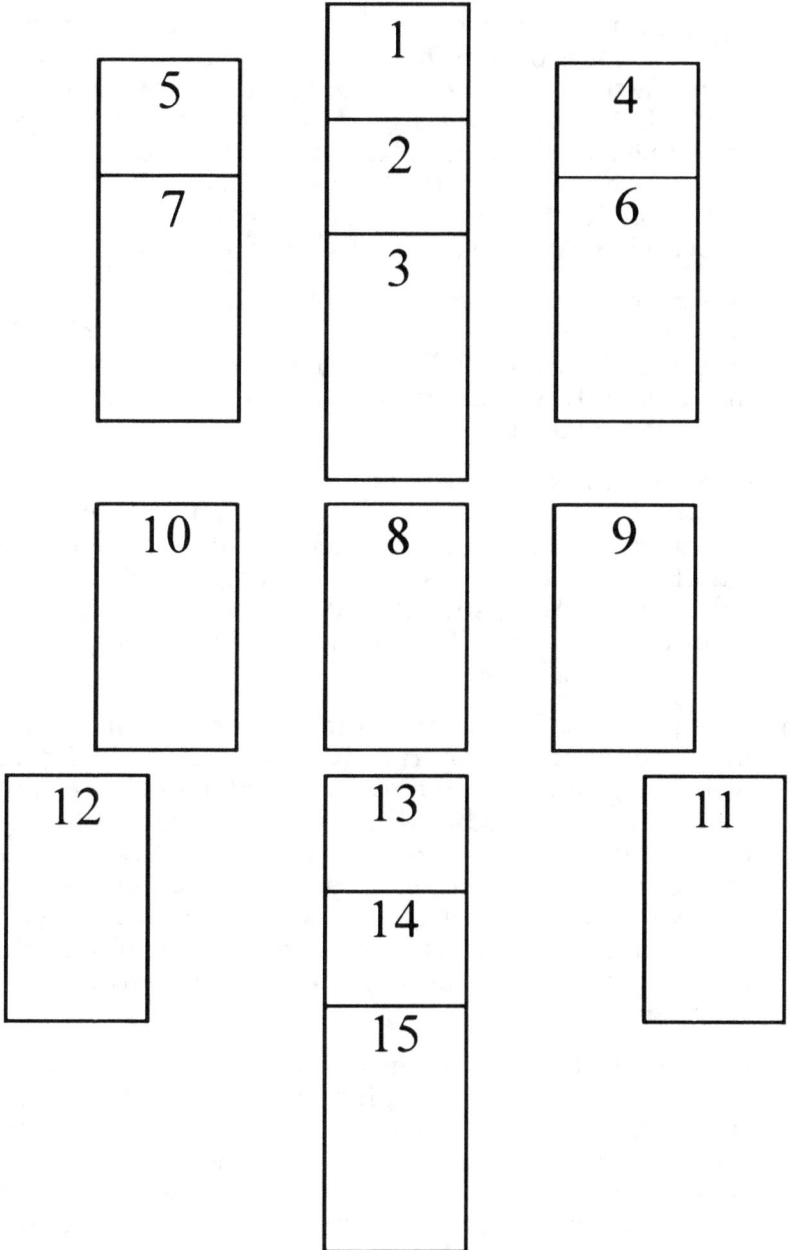

*Figure 5.1: The health layout*

## 5. Tarot as a healing tool: layouts

If something untoward shows in this position, and the physical symptoms presenting are not enough information to pinpoint the exact problem or what area of the head is affected, then narrow things down using a simple layout. To do that I use the Tree of Life layout and ask questions like 'is the problem infection?' 'is the problem inflammation?' and so on. Remember, the health reading only gives you an overview. After that, you need to focus in on specifics.

**The fourth position** shows us the solid energy going into the body. Anything that you are eating, drinking, smoking, or otherwise ingesting will show here, and the type of card that falls in this position will also indicate whether it is affecting you badly.

**The fifth position** shows the state of the emotions: how the person feels. Often the emotions can be very good indicators of what is going on deeper within the body. The emotions can drive the immune system, and when looking for a treatment ensure that it brings about favourable emotional energies. If a person is in physical pain, it will also show in this position.

**The sixth position** shows what the short-term or primary immune system is currently doing. If it is fighting something or it is in overdrive, it will show here. What we put into our bodies directly affects the front line of the immune system; hence this card sits directly under the 'solid energy' position. Look at the relations between the two cards: if an ingested substance (food, drugs etc) is contributing to, aggravating, or causing the illness, then both positions four and six will show aggravating or aggressive cards.

**The seventh position** shows the deeper immune system, and this is connected to the function of the thymus, an endocrine gland. The thymus prepares and trains T and B cells for a front-line attack on an intruder, and it is deeply affected by emotional wellbeing, which is why card seven sits beneath card five in this spread. This position also shows the secondary immune system that wraps up, locks up, or breaks down threats that have already been overcome.

When the querent is already on the winning side of an

## 5.4. The health layout

illness, the aggressive cards will often move from position six (primary immune response) to position seven. This is where disease threats are processed and put into 'sleep mode.' The person's emotional wellbeing will affect how well this process works, and if they have recently experienced terrible grief, this area of the immune system can become compromised. This position also tells us how our immune system is functioning. It indicates how well-balanced the immune responses are, and whether the body's T- and B-cells are being produced in the right quantities and are operating as they should, and are not attacking the body itself. (Regarding inflammatory diseases: when one is in active mode, it will often show in both immune positions. When the disease is dormant but has potential, it will show only in the seventh position.)

**The eighth position** shows the central core of the body, which houses the vital organs. If there is a problem with those organs, it will show here. If a major aggressive card falls in this position, then the reader needs to do further readings to see which specific organ has been affected.

**The ninth position** shows the male sexual organs, testosterone, and the bladder. Testosterone is also present in females, and if the reading is for a woman and a difficult card turns up in this position, then it will probably be necessary to look in more depth at her endocrine system and hormone balances. If they all look fine in separate readings, then a reading needs to be done to look at her hormonal response to being around males.

**The tenth position** shows the female sexual organs and the bladder. Again, males also have oestrogen in their bodies, so if the reading is for a male and a difficult card turns up here, check their hormone system. A difficult card here can also indicate the presence of a member of the opposite sex who is hormonally disruptive. So for example, if a woman magician is out-of-balance and a reading shows an aggressive card in the ninth position, it could either indicate a testosterone imbalance within her own body, or a male around her who is disrupting her health simply with his presence or energetic influence. This usually happens unconsciously, and it is the result of the many hormone signals our bodies put out—sometimes we can have a bad reaction to hormone signals coming from another person. Depending on where a woman is in her cycle, she can be attracted by male pheromones—but she can also be made aggressive by the presence of the same. In female magicians, this is far more pronounced than in the general population, depending on what streams of inner power and contacts they work with. So be aware of those possible dynamics when reading those positions: hormones are the dynamos that run our moods and emotions, and as such they have a powerful influence over everything that we do. The other thing that can show in these two sexual reproductive positions is bladder issues, so bear that in mind.

**The eleventh position** shows the digestive system, and it reveals how the large and small intestines are processing everything that came in at position four (food, etc). But be aware that a lot of magic can also be processed through the digestive system, particularly when we are given energy or information to take in. This area of the body can also be read in conjunction with position five (the emotions): there is a direct relationship between digestive health and mental and emotional health. For example, neurotransmitters like serotonin play a major part in mood, muscle health, and digestion.

**The twelfth position** tells us what is happening to us in our sleep. Many magicians put too much emphasis on controlling their dreams in order to have 'lucid dreams'. This is a mistake and it can interfere with true magical events that can happen in sleep, plus it also interferes with the body's own repair system that swings into action when we sleep.

Any magical intrusions of any real power will surface naturally in dreams, and dreams are also an opportunity for protective beings to warn us of impending trouble. Our sleep is also a time when our deeper spirit can partake of magical service, and it is unwise to interfere with the natural flow of our deeper selves. The dreams/sleep position is directly below the emotions and the deeper immune system in this layout, as they are all inexorably linked, and these cards can be read together to get a deeper understanding of what is happening in our subconscious, our brains, and our immune system. This position is also linked

## 5.4. The health layout

to positions one and two, and if disturbances show in positions one and two, and there is a volatile or difficult card in position twelve, then you are most likely looking at a magical attack, a difficult period of fate changes, or at least a magical disturbance. The quality of your sleep is very important to both your health and your strength, so pay good attention to what is going on in this position.

**The thirteenth position** looks at the 'structure and movement' system of the body, which means bone, muscle, and nerves. Any inflammatory reaction, central nervous system disturbance, or bone/muscle impact will show here. If there is a difficult card in this position and also in position three (head/brain), then you are more likely to be looking at a problem with nerve issues. If there are fiery cards in this position and in the eleventh position (digestion), then it may indicate an inflammatory disease active with roots in bacterial imbalance or inflammation in the small intestine.

**The fourteenth position** is the skin. The skin is the most externalized organ and also the biggest organ of our body. It is through the skin that the body can safely deposit toxins and dead matter, and process irritants: this mechanism keeps such problems away from vital organs, and also gives you a very obvious heads-up when there is a problem.

Issues with food sensitivity or allergy, recovery from viruses and infections, and reactions to magical power will all show on the skin: the skin is a very good weather indicator as to how our bodies are coping, and what they are coping with. If the magician is badly attacked and gets ill as a result, one of the healing objectives should be to bring that imbalance up to the surface to present itself on the skin. As soon as the rashes start to show, you know the healing process is working. Because of this mechanism, never be tempted to suppress rashes that appear; rather it is better to keep an eye on them and let them be. If it is an allergic reaction or a sensitivity reaction like eczema, find out the root cause and eliminate it if possible.

**The sixteenth position** tells us the immediate future of the body's health. If a damaging card turns up in this position, then work still has to be done to help to body come back into balance. Consider this card in relation to the time limit

## 5. Tarot as a healing tool: layouts

you put on the reading: if the reading looked three weeks ahead, and the card in position fifteen is a difficult one, then redo the reading to look at a span of six weeks, to see if the body just needs a bit more time to heal. If at six weeks the card in position fifteen (or other cards) is still difficult, then you need to reassess what action you are taking.

### 5.5 When to use the health layout

Use this layout when the body is showing obvious signs of distress after magical work, or if you body suddenly nosedives and you suspect that magic has been used. It is also a good layout to keep an eye on your general health, and can be used by energy healers to look at a client and get a deeper picture of what is going on inside their body.

Keep a record of the readings so that you can track recovery over time, but also so that you can spot potential longer-term problems that are not so apparent in the first readings. Often an imbalance in an area of the body starts like a grain of sand rubbing in your sock, but then grows over time to become a major issue. If that happens, you can go back over the readings to pinpoint the beginning of the problem and locate the area of the body that first went into decline. It also helps you to see how a particular body copes with problems: each body is slightly different and will have its own healing pattern. Through tracking various bodily reactions through readings, you can ascertain that body's own method of self-healing.

### 5.6 The endocrine layout

This layout (fig. 5.2) looks at some of the major endocrine glands in the body that are particularly affected by magic. They are master players in our health and close attention should be paid to them, particularly during long-term or powerful magical work. If the general health reading indicates an issue in the head (position three) and there are obvious signs in the body of endocrine disturbance (hormone swings, mood or appetite changes, thyroid issues, or an adrenal reaction without known cause (i.e. temperature swings), then it is time to look a bit closer at the endocrine system to see what is happening (and to go see a doctor).

When a magical attack or impact has gained access to the body, it will show up in this reading. If there is a major

## 5.6. The endocrine layout

disturbance in the body in general, it will most likely also show up here. The reason for doing this reading is to get more information: it is often unwise to attempt to influence the endocrine system directly unless you have medical training and a good idea of what you are doing. But this reading will give you a lot more information about how deep the effects of the magic or illness have gone, and also about how your own body operates.

Sometimes you need to deal directly with the endocrine system to bring about healing, and sometimes it is only necessary to be aware of which glands are struggling and adjust your life, diet and magic accordingly.

I will outline the functions of each gland below, but it would pay you dividends to do some further research, as any major magical hit will affect one or more of them at some point. No in-depth medical study is necessary, but a basic understanding of what these glands govern and affect is vital if you want to understand what is happening inside your body.

It is important to be aware that the activity of these glands tends to fluctuate a lot naturally, and if they go slightly out of balance, they are often able to rebalance themselves without any outside help. They also shift and change with age and with magical work. If you see a problem in one of the glands in a reading, don't automatically spring into action: just extend the time limits of the reading and see whether it will sort itself out.

Also be aware that not everything that shows up in this reading is caused by magic: usually these problems are caused by our food, our environment, things we spray on our bodies, situations we find ourselves in, and so forth. If you use the endocrine layout, work in tandem with the general health layout by having the health layout results written down so that you can look at both readings together. When a body has truly been hit by magic, then it is important to check the following key glands to see which ones are affected, and how they are coping.

**The first position** is the hypothalamus, which sits directly over the brainstem and is like the Hierophant of the body: it is the bridge between the nervous system and the endocrine system. It affects many vital core functions of the body, and from a magical perspective it governs our responses to energy intake, energy processing, identification (especially via smell) etc. The pituitary gland is often called the master gland, but the hypothalamus governs the pituitary: it is the CEO of the whole system.

## 5. Tarot as a healing tool: layouts

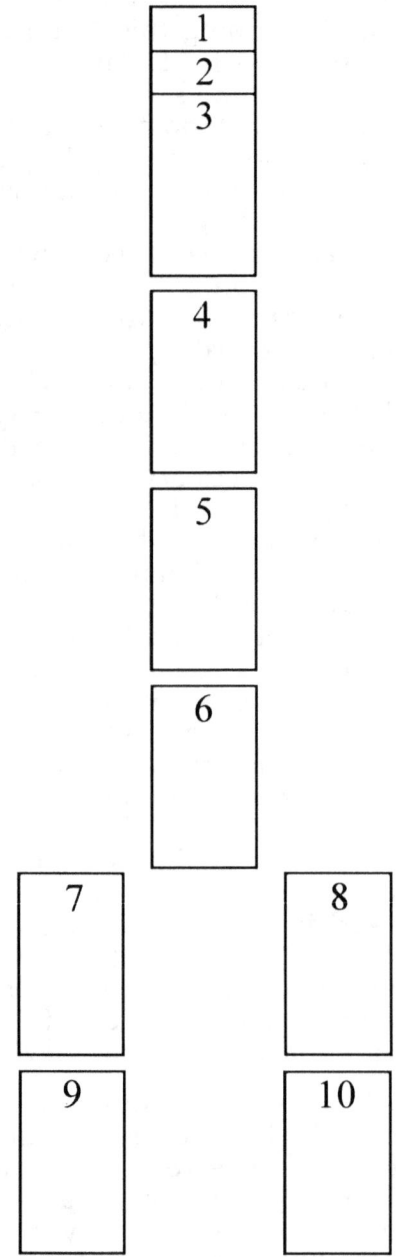

*Figure 5.2: The endocrine layout*

## 5.6. The endocrine layout

Most major Kabbalistic and high magic attacks will show up in this position, and if a being, magician, or angelic structure has gained access to your sphere, they too will show here. In such a case, the body would display a number of problems with sleep, appetite, temperature etc. If the attack shows up as attacking this gland but goes no further down the reading, then the body is already working to limit the invasion and push it out. If that is the case, then be careful not to interfere with the body's actions; rather it is better to look for ways to support it.

**The second position** is the pineal gland (also located in the brain) which is a gland that governs our seasonal and circadian rhythms, and connects us to the deeper tides of power that flow between the inner and outer worlds. If the magician is being affected by natural tides of power, then it will show here.

Treat such a discovery with some caution: being affected by these tides is perfectly normal. It only becomes an issue when it begins to actually to damage the body. We all have tidal slumps, but we generally recover quickly. But if you are being overwhelmed by a tidal wave of power, then it would most likely show here.

**The third position** is the pituitary gland (again located in the brain) which secretes the nine vital hormones that regulate homeostasis. The pituitary is part of a chain of glands (hypothalamic-pituitary-adrenal/HPA axis) that can be affected badly by magic: when the pituitary takes a hit, the impact can cascade through the body and cause all sorts of problems.

Often when there is a problem showing in the thyroid, adrenals, pancreas or ovaries, it tracks back to the pituitary gland and either stops there or goes back one step further to the hypothalamus. When the endocrine system has gone into disarray, even if such imbalance tracks all the way back to the hypothalamus, it is better to treat the pituitary if it is affected, rather than work directly with the hypothalamus. It is easier to make a mess by trying to treat the hypothalamus, as it is far more sensitive to deep treatments such as homeopathic endocrine sarcodes (see chapter on home-

## 5. Tarot as a healing tool: layouts

opathy). The pituitary is more robust, and will bounce back more easily if you make a mistake in energy treatment. The relationship between the hypothalamus and the pituitary is both medically and magically complex, so always consider these two glands together.

**The fourth position** is the thyroid gland, a good-sized butterfly-shaped gland which sits in the neck/throat with the larynx. It governs the processing and distribution of energy, and sets the hormone-sensitivity dials in other endocrine glands like the ovaries, testes, pancreas, etc. When a magician is working with a great deal of power, particularly if they are female, they tend to get hit in the thyroid.

If the magician goes into a decline after major work, and in particular if they are a woman, then it is wise to check this gland to see if it is operating properly. If it has taken a major hit, then the magician needs to visit a doctor to have their thyroid checked, and to get treated if the imbalance is strong enough to show up in blood tests.

If any hit was enough to affect the thyroid, but not enough to show in tests (or if the thyroid appears to be operating on the lower end of normal) then it is best to treat the gland with vitamins that have iodine in them, and direct visionary work on the gland. Just be careful with iodine as too much can adversely affect the health of the thyroid.

**The fifth position** is the thymus, which sits above the heart in the centre of the upper chest behind the breast bone. The thymus has two lobes that join in front of the trachea. The thymus is the wise old man of the immune system, which teaches immune cells how to fight and who to fight. From a magical perspective it is deeply connected to emotion and can be heavily impacted by grief. If a difficult card shows up in this position, and the cards above it are more or less normal, then any activity in this gland is more likely to be related to the immune system than a magical impact. If you have had a lot of grief, like a death or a divorce, then this gland needs a lot of care and support. This can be done using a visionary method of going and talking to the thymus by creating an imaginative image of a wise old man. This allows you to interface deeply with the gland and effect change.

**The sixth position** is the pancreas which produces insulin and sits under and behind the stomach. I have never noticed any particular engagement with this gland in magical terms. That does not mean there isn't one, only that I have not found any. The pancreas is involved in digestion and the processing sugar, so from a magical perspective it is a fuel processor. Just keep that in mind if you start to have energy problems, and difficult cards show up in this position.

**The seventh and eighth positions** are read together and are the adrenals. These sit over the kidneys on either side of your body and are your fight-or-flight system: they are chiefly a stress response team, though they also affect blood pressure and produce androgens.

The right adrenal is triangular in shape, and the left is half-moon shaped. I mention the difference because I have noticed in readings that each adrenal gland acts very differently from its partner: in a magical attack one will take up the battle, while the other becomes a watchman. It is important to keep an eye on them so that they do not burn out, and if they are showing signs of strain in a reading, then it would be a good idea to back off any heavy inner work for a while to give them a rest.

Sometimes you can detect a clever sneak magical attack by doing a reading if you suspect something is going on: it will show the engagement of one of the adrenals, as they function as lookouts as well as providing the first line of defence.

**The ninth and tenth positions** are the ovaries or testes, and this is where any possible parasite infestation will show, as will children hanging around waiting to be conceived, etc. If a magical attack is directed at a person's fertility or relationship, then it will most likely show here.

## 5.7 The four-directional layout: power incoming

This layout (fig. 5.3) is good for seeing what is being aimed directly at you from the inner worlds, be it tides, attacks, contacts, or something else. This layout describes the body itself and its general energetic status, and then goes on to show inner energies coming out of the four magical directions. It ends with the final

## 5. Tarot as a healing tool: layouts

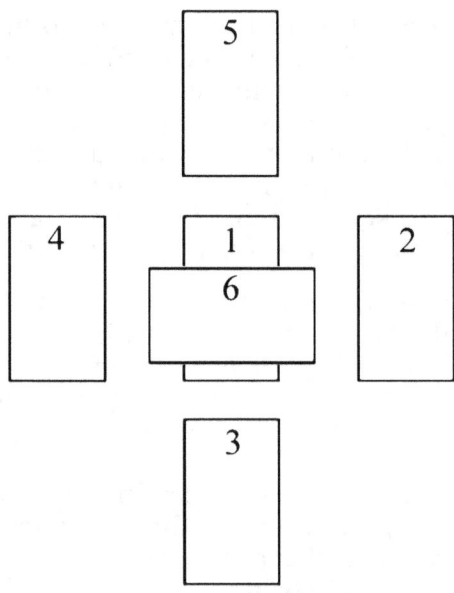

*Figure 5.3: The four-directional layout*

card crossing the body, which shows what power or person the querent is currently engaged with.

The four directional layout is extremely flexible and can be used for all sorts of different questions. It is rooted in directional qualities, seasons, time, and types of magic. For a health reading, you can use it to look at magical attacks or magical tides of power to discern what type of magic is being used or is flowing around a person. Don't always assume something is an attack – a successful attack is far less likely than, for example, a physical rebound from a magical working.

Use this layout in conjunction with the others to get specifics regarding what type of magic is being used, or what magical power lies behind energies or contacts, or to track the progress of an attack or magical impact.

**The first position** tells us about the body. If the body itself is ill or out of balance, it will show in this position.

**The second position** tells us what energies or magic are coming from the magical direction of east. This would be forms of ritual magic that use utterance, air or swords, like Kabbalah for instance, Western Mysteries magic, or any other similar system. It will show magic that is aimed at silencing a voice or stopping communication. It will also show new attacks that are just coming in.

**The third position** tells us about the magical use of fire, fire temple magic, or any magic that conjures fire or heat or is aimed at making a person ill. It also represents the pinnacle of a magical attack.

**The fourth position** tells us of emotive magic or magic that is water-based. If an attack is aimed at a person's relationships or fertility, it will show here. It also shows magic that is near completion.

**The fifth position** tells us of tribal, witchcraft or earth-based magic, or magic aimed at the bones or the body's structure. It is also the position of 'passing away'—magic that is now fading.

**The sixth position** tells us of our relationships, and depending on the question, can show the magician's actual relationships or the powers and people they are currently interacting with.

## 5.8 The Desert/Inner Landscape layout

I designed this layout out of the sheer need for more information. It is very versatile and can be applied in a number of ways depending on what information you need: focusing on your question and also your application of the layout will direct the reading to the layer of consciousness that you are trying to observe. It can be used to look at a person's inner landscape, or a person's outer life, or to examine a space, building, lodge or magical group to see what dynamics are currently in play and what will be the result of the current situation.

In terms of health, it is best employed to look at a person's inner landscape. Through the various positions we learn what current fate or path dynamics are in play, what are the problems to be overcome, what powers are coming out of the inner worlds, and what powers are present in the home, the dreams, and so on.

If for example a magician's health reading shows problems in the first and second position, then it is time to do a Desert layout to look at their inner landscape. If after doing the Desert

## 5. Tarot as a healing tool: layouts

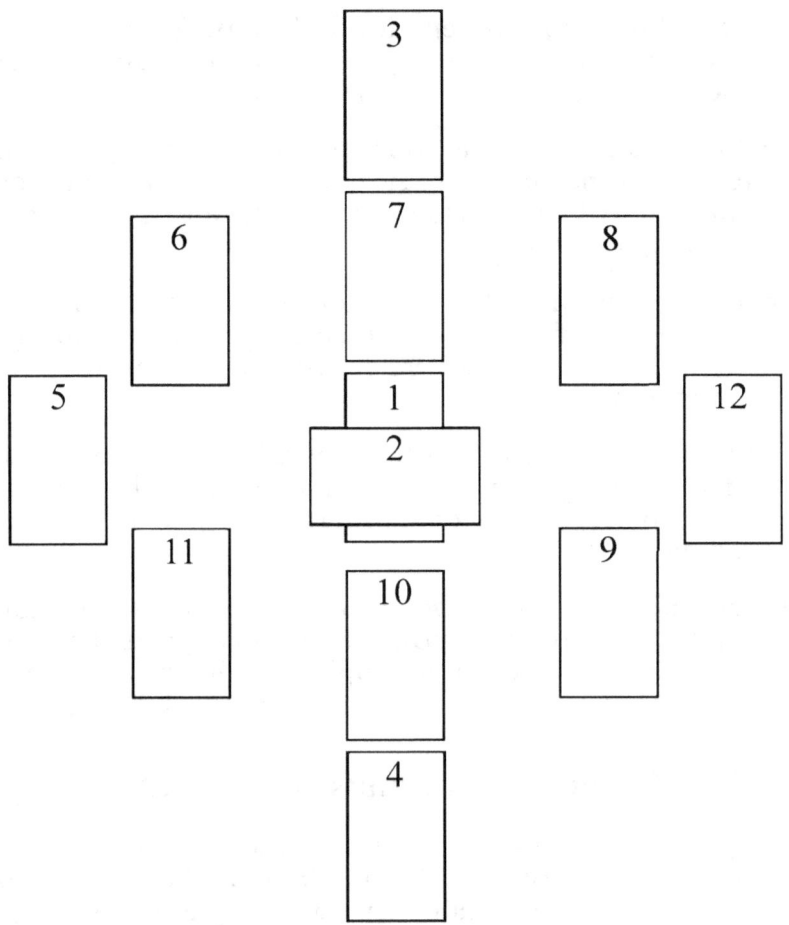

*Figure 5.4: The Desert/Inner Landscape layout*

layout further information is needed as to the nature of the inner power in question, then use the four-directional reading described above to look at the inner power in detail. The Desert layout gives situational information, and the four directional reading shows power sources and shapes.

**The first position** is the body. It tells us what state the body is in with regards to health and vitality.

**The second position,** which crosses the first, tells us what power or people dynamics we are currently dealing with.

## 5.8. The Desert/Inner Landscape layout

**The third position** tells us what is coming in the long-term future, a pattern that is still being formed in the stars. If a resolution is coming but will take some time to arrive, then that will show here; however if the problem will be prolonged, that will also be indicated here.

**The fourth position** shows us what has already passed away down into the depths, which will not be revisiting us anytime soon.

**The fifth position** shows us the gate to the past: this is the threshold of what is now in the immediate past. Whatever occupies this position has the potential to return at some point in the future, but for the moment can be considered past.

**The sixth position** describes the pattern of fate or action that is currently playing out: for example a struggle, a cycle of magical work, a period of renewal, etc. This is the path you are currently on, unless you do something to change that path's direction. The fate path indicated in position six is not your overall life time fate, but the current cycle of lesser fate/events that are presently active.

**The seventh position** shows hardships or difficulties that must be overcome. These are not warnings to be avoided, but show the process of how the healing can come about – what needs to be pushed through, endured or waited out.

**The eighth position** shows what is coming directly into your landscape from the inner worlds. All magical attacks, inner contacts, work programs, inner support, deities etc. will show here.

**The ninth position** shows the effect your home, family and surroundings are having on your health. For example, if there is a haunting, a bad energy, or difficulty in the home environment that is making you ill or tired, it will show here. It can also be a position to indicate where the reproductive hormone system is having problems.

**The tenth position** describes what is falling away or starting to go into decline: if you have defeated something, or if something is starting to leave your body or fate path, it will show here. It is travelling towards the gate of the past and will finally vanish into the depths. If, however, you do not meet the challenges that appear in the seventh position, then any difficulties shown here in the tenth position will come right back to challenge you until you get the message.

**The eleventh position** represents the dreams and sleep. This position tells you what your deeper unconscious mind is dealing with, and what is happening to you in your sleep.

**The twelfth position** shows the way ahead, and tells you the immediate outcome to your question. For a longer-term outcome, look to position three.

The Desert layout is very elegant in how it works and has many different applications depending on the question and context. It is the spread I use the most, and whereas the health reading gives you an overview of what is going on in the body, the Desert reading gives an overview of fate paths and magical events that are going on in the magician's inner and outer life.

If you need a straight yes or no answer to a question, then the Tree of Life layout will facilitate a straight forward answer. I use the Tree of Life spread in the context of magical health when I need to choose a treatment style (i.e. is this treatment the best way forward, yes or no?), and once I have an idea of the best way forward, then I will go back to the health reading and see how that treatment would play out in the body.

## 5.9 The Tree of Life layout

The Tree of Life layout (fig. 5.5) is another versatile spread and can be applied to almost any question. As with most things in life though, its greater versatility comes at the cost of detail. When you use the Tree of Life layout for a health reading, it must be interpreted in terms of the body, otherwise it is useless.

What follows is a quick guide to using the Tree of Life positions for health. The interpretations listed for this layout are specific to health readings. When using the Tree of Life layout for wider subject matter, the interpretations of the positions change somewhat.

**The first, second, and third positions** are read together, and show us what the story is about.

**The fourth position** reveals what is happening to the body that is active (this position is good regardless of whether it is a bad card or not).

## 5.9. The Tree of Life layout

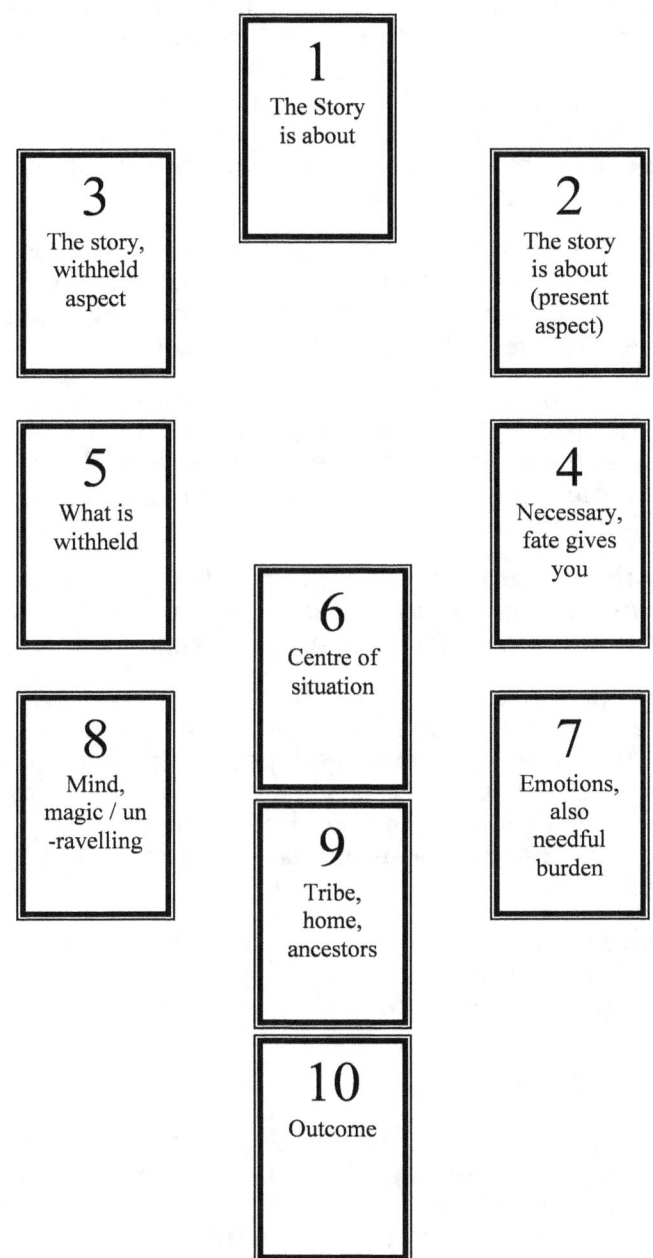

*Figure 5.5: The Tree of Life layout*

## 5. Tarot as a healing tool: layouts

**The fifth position** shows what is withheld. This means what is being *held back* from the body. If regeneration falls in this position, for example, then they body cannot regenerate until something else has been released or resolved (usually indicated in position six). If a fiery or destructive card falls in position five, however, then the body has been able to overcome whatever it was fighting.

**The sixth position** represents the centre of the situation, so for example if the magician had been hit by a lot of power and was ill, you would expect to see the Tower, the Ten of Wands, or the Ten of Swords in this position.

**The seventh position** describes the heart and emotions (including physical pain). Pay attention to what shows up in this position, as the emotions are key indicators of the balance of energetic health, and they play a major part in any recovery from illness.

**The eighth position** is the mind and brain. If there is a problem in the central nervous system, it will show here. This position can also show any magical aggravation.

**The ninth position** represents the reproductive system and dreams: it can be read as either. How you interpret this position (the Moon) largely depends on what you want to know and what you are asking. So if someone was having problems with their sleep or dreams, then it will show here. But it can also be a position that indicates genetic/ancestral conditions.

**The tenth position** gives you your answer or outcome. The preceding nine positions will have told you how this outcome will come about.

## 5.10 Shuffling

How you approach shuffling the cards can be just as important as any other aspect of working with tarot. Everyone develops their own shuffling technique, but there are some points to consider in order to make the shuffling successful.

One key factor is to ensure that you are fully focused on the question in hand as you shuffle. Do not be distracted by talking, or allow your mind to wander: keep the question foremost in your mind as you work the cards. One good method for doing that is to work with your eyes closed. As you shuffle, think about the question and imagine you are searching for something through a 'mist'. Use your inner vision and imagination to create the sensation of trying to 'pierce a veil'.

As you develop your technique, you will find that after the initial shuffle, your hand action begins to slow down so that the cards are placed more precisely in their order. Once everything is in the right position you will feel them 'lock' in place. The accuracy of a reading relies on the focus of intention you hold as you work the cards.

Once your deck is ready, work from the top of the pile and place each card out. Once you have become accustomed to working with cards, you may find that the answer you were looking for seeps into your mind even before you lay the cards out. It is as if you get a preview of what is coming. Not all readers have this experience, but for those with a strong natural ability, the flavour of the reading often emerges in the reader's mind before the cards are laid out.

## 5.11 Cleaning hands and decks

Once the readings are finished, it is advisable to go and wash your hands with soap. If it has been a difficult reading, or if the reading was used to look at difficult, dangerous or unhealthy situations, then it is a good idea to put some salt in the cup of your hand before adding soap and water. This will break any energetic ties and will also clean off the 'sticky' energetic residue that can sometimes accumulate during readings.

Depending on how often you use the deck (and always after very difficult readings) it can be a good idea to clean the deck itself. This can be done by 'bathing' the deck in the smoke from frankincense resin burned on charcoal, or by putting the deck in a plastic bag, pouring in dry salt, and giving it a good shake.

This limits the lifespan of the deck itself, but it is more important to stay clean than to have a grubby favourite deck for years. This is why for most readings it is wiser to use a common, simple deck that can be easily and affordably replaced on a regular basis. My deck usually lasts me about a year before I have to replace it, and I use my deck regularly.

Store your deck in a box, and keep it away from children, pets etc. Wrapping the deck in a cloth and using a cloth for layouts also helps to limit any unhealthy energy residue from being left

## 5. Tarot as a healing tool: layouts

behind, and also it helps to stop the deck from getting dirty. The cloth should be washed regularly.

## 5.12 Summary

The key to working with these layouts is to be very clear with your questions, and to be clear in your mind about what the layout looks like. In the early days of working with a new layout, I find it easier if I draw the layout on a piece of cloth and put the cards out on that.

It is also important to be able to interpret what you are seeing. Keep it simple, and most of the time you will find it is the most obvious answer: for example in the Rider-Waite deck the Ten of Wands/Fire shows a man with a bundle of sticks on his back. In a health reading it is a burden of fire—a fever or massive inflammation. In a reading to do with magic it still means a burden of fire, but this time a magical one. This is what I mean when I say that you should read simply, but in context.

In the next chapter, Part Two of Diagnostic Tarot, we will look at these layouts in terms of interpretation, using some examples so that you can get an idea of how it all pulls together. In a session you may need to use several different layouts with different questions, or sometimes you can get all the information you need in one simple layout.

The only limits in tarot are the ones you put upon yourself. The cards themselves are not magical; they are simply a vocabulary that can be used both by your own consciousness and also for communication between inner beings and yourself—remember that!

For the next chapter, have a copy of the Rider-Waite deck to hand, and map out the various layouts so that you can work with me: lay the cards out, and follow my interpretations of the sample readings.

Chapter Six

# *Tarot as a healing tool: interpretation*

## 6.1 Reading the signs

In this chapter we will look at interpretations via a series of readings around magical health issues. Have a Rider Waite Tarot deck to hand, and also the maps of the spreads so that you can lay out the cards for the readings and follow the interpretations. Note: I do not use reversals in tarot readings; I get the negative information I need via the layout positions and the cards themselves.

Always keep a record of your readings, so that you can refer back to them once an incident has occurred: after having experienced something you predicted in a reading, going back and looking again at the reading will teach you a great deal about how the cards operate for you as an individual reader.

To demonstrate how to use the layouts, I have chosen to look at the health and magical situation of a well-known magician who died at the age of fifty five after a long magical career. The magician I have chosen to look at is Dion Fortune. The reason I chose her, besides the fact that her life and work are pretty well known, is that she was involved in the Magical Battle of Britain during World War Two, and I always had a suspicion that this work contributed to her death.

Although many magicians were involved in that battle, DF took it personally and felt she was battling to save her beloved country. The approach that they took was over-structured and did not allow the deeper powers within the land to surface and be used. Instead the burden fell upon the magicians who were working, and many paid a difficult price for their service.

The group, which was directed by DF, drew upon mythical patterns of the Arthurian legends, the Grail legends, Christian mystical forms, and angelic magical structures. Because they drew upon mythic patterns that had become romanticized and were not fully of this land, they were unable to draw on the vast magical resources that lie dormant within the land of Britain.

## 6. Tarot as a healing tool: interpretation

But we are all of our time; they drew on what they knew best and worked very hard at it. It is important to remember, as we look back and pick apart their actions, that we are all of our time. It is easy to criticize in retrospect, but they sacrificed a great deal in their efforts to protect the sacred land.

I am sure that in the future, we magicians of today will also be criticized for the methods, filters and structures that we use. If that happens, then we have done our job successfully. Such insight from future magicians means that we laid our foundations well for them to stand upon, and that magic developed and matured within the generations that followed us.

I started the reading session with the assumption that it was the Battle of Britain that killed Dion Fortune in 1946 (she died of advanced leukaemia). After doing a few different readings and looking at her health from different angles, a more complicated story started to emerge. The following readings use the various layouts to look at her situation from different angles. One reading would lead to another question, which gives you the chance to see how diagnostic enquiry can work.

Lay the cards out for yourself, and look at the overall feel and picture of the readings. Before you start to interpret, just take time to look at the overall spread, and let the images on the cards tell you a story.

### 6.2   Diagnostic reading

The first spread to use in any magical diagnostic heath enquiry is the health spread itself. I thought a lot about how to phrase the initial query: we want to see the effects of the magical work on her health (or not). So I decided to start with a broad picture of the last five years before her death.

Because this covers a lot of time, it will give us a wide view of the major dynamics that were happening within and around her body. The further back you stand to 'snap' your picture, the more you will see the major influences, but the less you will see of the details.

I expected to see a strong, healthy reading with a sudden downward spiral before her death. It has always been said by her organization (Society of the Inner Light) that she was very vital and healthy right up until shortly before her death, and that she suddenly became ill after the war ended. Interestingly, the health readings show a different picture altogether.

## 6.2. Diagnostic reading

With the Health layout in front of you and using the Rider Waite Deck, place the cards out in the order shown in fig. 6.1.

**The first card**, which shows what is coming out of the inner worlds, is the **nine of swords**. This card represents suffering or defeat (and I also read this card as a 'sneaky attack' or aggression that is cloaked or unseen). In its position, it immediately alerted me to an inner impact of some kind.

**The second card**, the **six of wands**, represents victory and is sitting in the position of her inner landscape. This shows the victorious conclusion of a battle won: the successful leader. Appearing in her inner landscape means the pattern for that victory was already formed from an inner perspective, and was starting to externalize itself. In magical terms, she was successful in battle.

**The third card** is the **King of Swords**. In a health reading this card is often a warning where the body is trying to guard its precious resources: it focuses right down to necessary functions only. This sort of card in this position tells me that something in her head or neck was under threat. That could be her brain, sinuses, ears, eyes, nose, mouth or thyroid. I would guess it was her thyroid, judging from her shape and the way she did magic. (If you really needed to know exactly what is being affected, then you would do Tree of Life spread to look at the brain, thyroid, sinus etc. individually.) Bear in mind at this point in the reading we are looking at a five year period, not just the last few months of her life. So the pattern of problems her body struggled with was apparent a few years before she died.

**The fourth card** is the **six of swords**. In the fourth position this can be read as a change in diet/intake for the better: it looks possible that her diet changed or she started to take something (herbs etc) in an attempt to improve her health.

**The fifth card**, which is the position of emotions, is the **four of swords** which is withdrawing, rest or seclusion. It tells me that her emotions were starting to withdraw, and that she would have felt tired and numb.

From a health perspective, if you look back to the card in position three (king of swords) you will see that the brain was under stress. This could be related to the beginnings

## 6. Tarot as a healing tool: interpretation

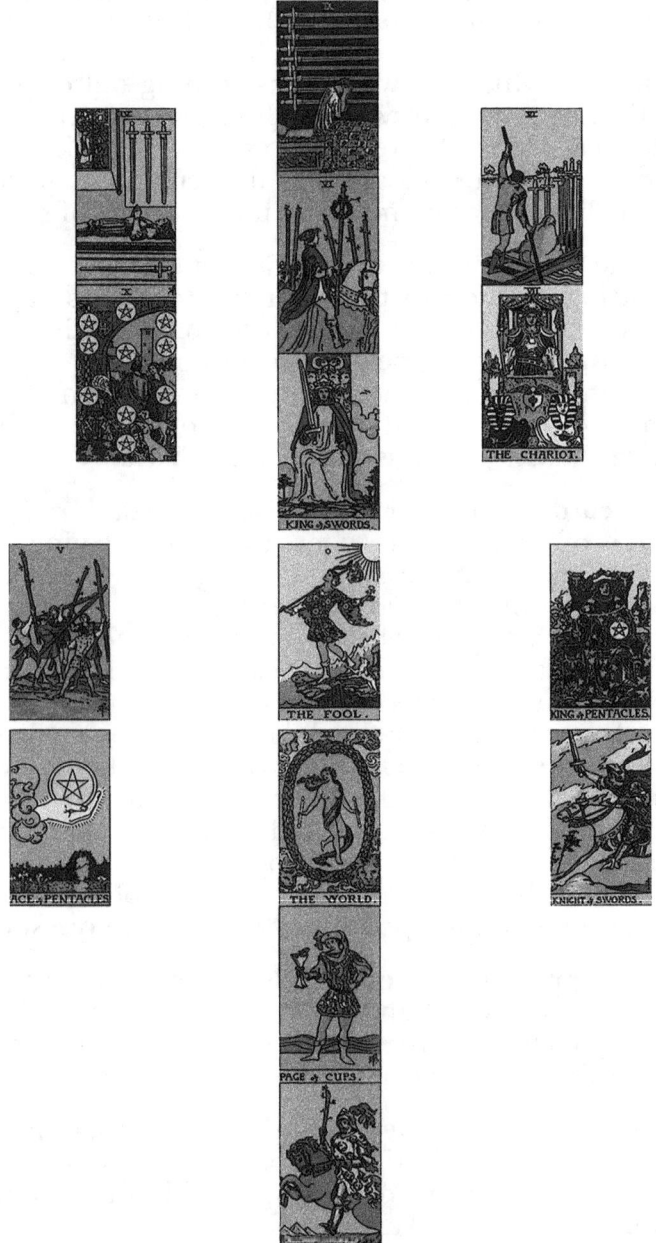

*Figure 6.1: Health reading: Dion Fortune's last five years.*

## 6.2. Diagnostic reading

of her leukaemia, or to the menopause, stress or diet.

When the brain is out of balance, the first signs of it are often changes in personality or the emotions being deadened. The same picture can be seen in clinical depression, PTSD, the early stages of multiple sclerosis, and other neurological illnesses that directly affect the central nervous system. The way to try and establish the root cause of these deadened emotions is to look at the other cards in key areas. Let's see what else we find.

**The sixth card** is the **Chariot**. It is a major card, and it shows the immune system being galvanized in a big way. This is not really a good card to find in this position for a five-year reading: it is too powerful and too active for such a long period of time, and it suggests that the immune system is running out of control.

**The seventh card** is the **ten of pentacles**. The ten of pentacles is a lot of substance i.e. it can indicate too much of something. (For example, in the bones/nerves position it can indicate too much calcium.) In the seventh position, which is the long-term immune system, it could represent a clogging-up, or a pattern of overgrowth. I do not know of any connection between the thymus (the gland which governs this position) and overgrowth/cancer, but it is an odd card to find here.

When you come up against something like this in a reading that you do not understand, simply take note, go away and read up around the issue, or watch to see what happens.

**The eighth card**, which represents the vital organs and also the vital force, is **the Fool**. The internal organs are disordered and the vital force is literally 'stepping off the cliff'. In a health reading, the Fool represents a lack of wisdom or knowledge about the position's correct function—that is, something is just not happening. Another way to read that is that something is 'empty'.

**The ninth card**, which represents the male force, is the **King of Pentacles**. In women this implies the influence of her 'male' hormones (such as testosterone) or a male contact. This card needs to be read in conjunction with other layouts to clarify its meaning. It does show up in later readings for

## 6. Tarot as a healing tool: interpretation

DF, so we will come to the potential meaning of this card later.

**The tenth card** is the **five of swords**, which is an argumentative card. For a woman, this position refers to her hormones, and this particular card indicates disturbance and argument in her hormone system. This is not unusual for a woman of her age, as she would have been in the midst of menopause. So overall it is not necessarily an indication of bad health; rather it shows that her endocrine system was in a state of flux and needed some support.

**The eleventh card** is the **Knight of Swords**. This position is the lower part of the digestive system (large and small intestine, bowel etc.) and would indicate that her small intestines were fighting some infection or bacterial overgrowth (if it was the knight of fire, we would more likely be looking at inflammation or an allergic reaction).

This could potentially connect back to the cards in the third position (brain) and the fifth position (emotion). Why? Because a bacterial overgrowth or an inflammation of the small intestines has a direct effect on the health of the brain and nervous system, via the development of neurotransmitters in the small intestine along with the absorption of vital nutrients. If this system is disrupted, and the gut becomes leaky or inflamed, then the nervous system begins to suffer depletion. The other possible option for this card in this position is the notion that she may have been processing magical power or a contact through her digestive system.

**The twelfth card**, which is the realm of sleep and dreams, is the **Ace of Pentacles**. This card can indicate a 'plug' or 'block' when it appears in health readings, and it tells us that her sleep and dreams were blocked in some way. This could also relate back to either the health of the brain or to a magical block. We have some anecdotal evidence from her colleagues that in the last few years of her life she seemed to suffer from a loss of inner contact at some level. While the Society of the Inner Light (her magical organization) has vigorously denied these reports, this reading suggests that there may have been some truth to them. Looking at the overall reading, I suspect the blocking happened naturally as the body attempted to cling on to whatever

## 6.2. Diagnostic reading

vital force was left. When we are ill, sometimes we find ourselves blocked from deeper inner work as the body's self-defence mechanism kicks in.

**The thirteenth card** is the **World**, a powerful trump card. This tells us that her bones and nerves were in good health. This would seem to contradict our hypothesis that a problem in her small intestine lay at the root of issues with her emotions, sleep and brain. If that hypothesis was correct, we would have expected to see damage to the peripheral nerves, or at least some level of inflammation.

Instead, it takes us back to the very first card, which shows defeat coming from the inner worlds. So we start to see a picture of a magical impact that hit the brain (king of swords) and affected the emotions (four of swords). The aggressive power of the impact was channelled through the small intestine and bowel in an attempt to process it safely. It did, however, prove overwhelming for her system.

**The fourteenth card** is the **Child of Cups**. This is the position of the skin, and it is a benign card. So the battle that was going on deep within her system did not exteriorize through her skin. If it had, she would have had a better fighting chance.

**The fifteenth card** is the **Knight of Wands**. This fire card in health readings often shows a fight with something fiery like inflammation, radiation or acute infection that the body is not fighting well. These court cards can sometimes indicate a specific illness that is aggressive and quick-moving. It shows up in her later readings, too, and I think it indicates the Leukaemia itself.

After I had finished this reading, I sat back and looked at the overall picture, and bearing in mind that it covered a span of five years, it told me that the battle that waged within her was long-standing (and therefore not the Battle of Britain), and caused by magical inner-world events or contacts. I began to suspect that the Battle of Britain was not so much the cause of her illness as the straw that broke the camel's back.

Because the reading spanned five years, I had expected to see relatively benign cards littering most of the reading, with the aggression or battle showing its effect only in the last few cards. But the victory in the inner landscape told me that while she

## 6. Tarot as a healing tool: interpretation

was successful in her magical battle, her body was already falling apart around it. And of course, we will never know exactly *what* she was fighting in those years before she died.

Just a word of caution here for when you do your own health readings: this reading has a long time-span, so only the most powerful events show and the cards must be read in context of that power. If this reading was for a span of four weeks, I would be more inclined to say that the person was facing a health crisis, but not such a serious one. We all have health problems at some point or other. If I saw a four-week reading like this for someone, I would then open the time span out to six months. Usually, in such circumstances the crisis vanishes in the second reading and becomes a minor issue indicated by one or two cards: the severity of a problem must be read within the context of the time-span of the reading.

When I had finished looking at this reading, I decided to focus in and get more information on the first card that appeared: the nine of swords. That seemed to be the catalyst or main indicator of cause. So I asked about the nine of swords. My question was, 'what is this nine of swords about for her?' The answer was as shown in fig. 6.2.

**The first card** represents the body itself. The **Knight of Wands** (Fire) showed up in most of her readings, and seemed to symbolize the leukaemia pattern. Having a fiery, energetic and immature card like this representing the body of woman of menopausal age is not a good sign. You might expect to see this in the body of a young energetic person who is full of beans (and hormones) and is still maturing. But for a person in her late forties or early fifties and beyond, it indicates something 'burning through' the body, something aggressive—and something immature and dangerous. It is interesting to note that leukaemia is an issue with immature white blood cells running amok, which makes the knight of fire a good depiction of such a disease.

**In the East** was the **King of Pentacles**, another card that repeatedly showed up. It indicates an inner contact, possibly ancestral, and one which may be connected to her work with the land. Because it is 'outside' her body but represented by a human form, it is most likely to be an inner contact, i.e. an inner adept or ancestor.

## 6.2. Diagnostic reading

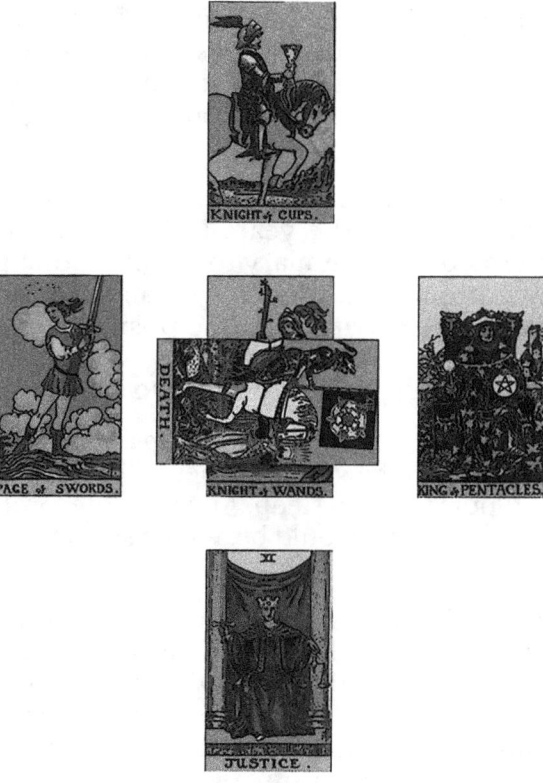

*Figure 6.2: Four-directional reading: 'What is this nine of swords about for her?'*

**In the South** was the trump **Justice**, which I took to be her battle for the land. The south is the position where you would expect to see volatile magic that causes inflammation and aggressive disease: the magic of the south is an extreme fire temple magic, and is often associated with war, absolute leaders, the fire of aggressive madness, and extreme testosterone powers. This was what she was fighting.

It also collates with what was showing in her inner landscape, which was victory: she and those who worked with her won the battle from an inner point of view, and she brought Justice/balance back to the land. Another interpretation of this card in this position would be that she was personally given justice: through her battle or her illness,

## 6. Tarot as a healing tool: interpretation

something was brought back into balance. Keep in mind that the tarot trump Justice does not necessarily relate to a modern Western sense of justice; rather it is more akin to the laws of Ma'at which is all about restoring balance.

**In the West** we see the **Page of Swords**. Pages have always been a nightmare for me to read, as they can mean so many things. Over the years I have narrowed this card down in my own vocabulary to mean writing projects and sneaky communications. I am guessing that in her sphere, it represents her writing. In the position of the West we have the creative depths, dreams, visions and so on; plus she identified very strongly with the sea and its mysteries.

**In the North** was the **Knight of Cups**: a romantic male connection falling away from her. The North takes things away and puts them to sleep. Another interpretation of this card in this position would be a male spirit waiting in death for her.

**The final card,** which crosses the querent, was **Death**: so already the relationship with death had started and she was walking the path towards her own death. Usually when Death appears in this position it marks the end of something, which could be a relationship, an illness, a way of life, etc. It is always a situation that cannot be gone back on. Her divorce from Penry Evans was in 1939, before the span of this reading, and seeing as I was specifically looking at physical and magical health, I discounted the death in this position to be her marriage. For her, Death was literal, and it was in her pattern up to five years before she died.

At this point, the conclusion I came to was that the nine of swords which figured in her health reading was neither an 'attack,' nor a simple illness; rather it was an impact from her magical work that ignited something already present in her body. Unfortunately for her, it was extreme in its conclusion.

Usually magical impacts tend to just bring out latent imbalances so that we can deal with them. Dion Fortune was unlucky. Plus there is the dynamic that the more power you work with, the more likely the fallout will be spectacular in its presentation. I became more curious about the implications that her pattern of death was already in place five years before she died. Now I wanted to know, how far back did that pattern go?

## 6.2. Diagnostic reading

I decided to do another reading to look at her vital force and see what her resources were like ten years before the Magical Battle of Britain started. That would potentially give me more idea of what happened, why it happened, and maybe how it happened.

My question was: 'what was the state of her vital force ten years before the Battle of Britain?' I decided to use a Tree of Life spread (fig. 6.3), as I wanted a straight answer. Again, bear in mind that this is a health reading, not a life situation reading: the cards must be read as indicators of physical, mental, emotional and spiritual health.

**The first card**, the **seven of wands**, clearly shows DF already struggling to stay on her feet. Because the question was about her vital force, this is what the reading is looking at, rather than her overall health. Ten years before the magical Battle of Britain, her vital force was already fighting to stay intact. At this point she was still on the upper hand of the struggle, but it was a struggle nonetheless. The slump in vital force comes to many magicians, and is often the herald of an initiatory illness.

Unfortunately for DF, the cultural attitude of the time was to 'soldier on, chin up, and don't give in to the slump.' For a magician faced with a deficit of vital force, that is the worst possible attitude to take (see summary).

**The second card** is **Strength**. This is her overall strength: her strong constitution and focused mind were keeping her going, and up to that point were holding back the tidal wave that would ultimately sweep her off her feet.

**The third card** is the **Child of Swords**, which probably indicates her writing: she was battling to keep the work going, but it was beginning to be a struggle (position three, Binah, is the negative aspect of the 'story is about'). Strangely enough it was probably the writing that kept her going for so long.

**The fourth card** is the **Hermit**: something happened around this time (1936) that made her re-evaluate everything energetically at a deep level. This interpretation is further strengthened by the appearance of the Wheel of Fortune in position six: the centre of the reading. A major change was happening on a deep level in her health and vitality.

## 6. Tarot as a healing tool: interpretation

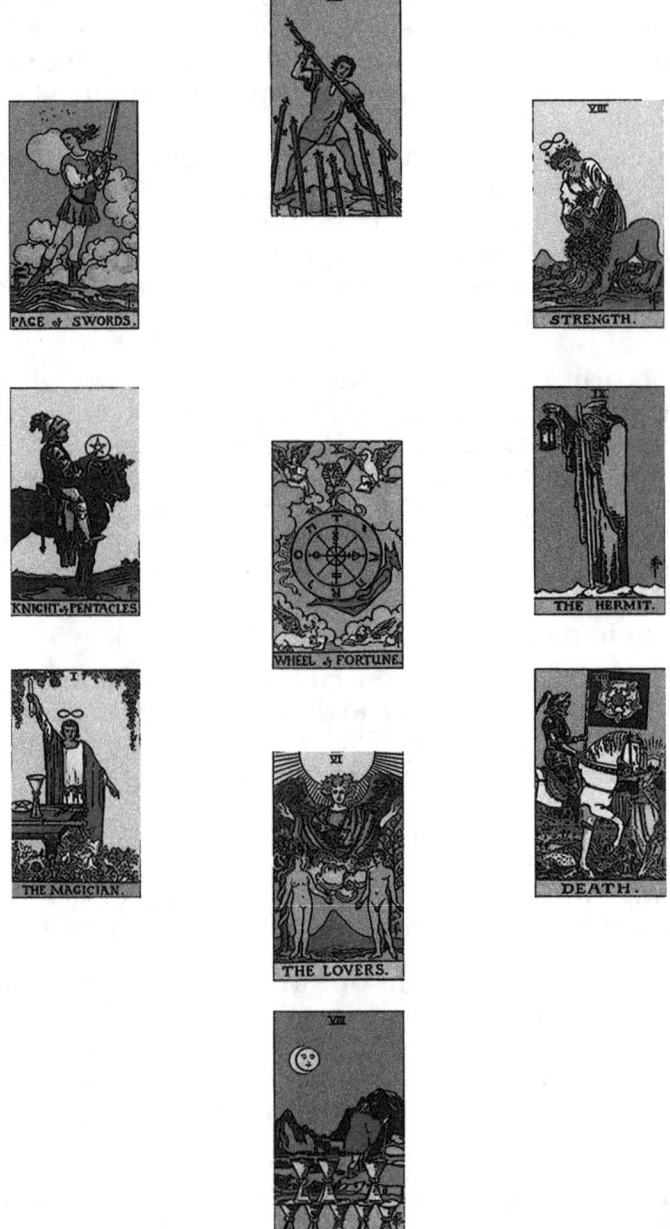

*Figure 6.3: Tree of Life reading: 'what was the state of her vital force ten years before the Battle of Britain?'*

## 6.2. Diagnostic reading

Positions four, five and six are often read together: they are the scale's two pans, and the fulcrum in the centre.

**The fifth card,** in the position of withholding, is the **Knight of Pentacles.** I would read this as a change in direction of her work from the mythic Arthur (or the loss of an ancestral health pattern) to something deeper. The reason I assume this has to do with writing, even though it is a health reading, is that her magical writing had a direct influence on her energy and vitality. Whatever that Knight was in position five, it was connected to this massive shift in energy (Wheel) and a period of introspection and/or energetic re-evaluation (Hermit).

**The seventh card** is **Death.** This is a common combination when someone has low vital force: their emotions deaden in a way that you also see with post-traumatic stress disorder. If the brain is under too much magical strain, the loss of emotions is often a major indicator that things are not going well. This card also supports what we saw in the health layout regarding the brain and emotions.

**The eighth card** is the **Magician.** This represents her working magically through the use of her mind (visionary magic). So even though her vital force was already under threat, she was still working powerfully (the Magician trump in the eighth position is about as strong as you can get).

**The ninth card** is the **Lovers:** her vital force was working strongly from a sexual point of view, and in this position (the Moon, Imagination) it would indicate that she was highly sexed at this time of her life, but only in the use of her mind. Her use of the mind for sex was most likely a reaction to the heavy Victorian mindset she was born into. But with such experimentation came a lot of parasitical risks that could have contributed to her energy depletion.

**The tenth card,** and the most important one as it gives us our answer, is the **eight of cups.** This card is about moving away and moving on. I do not use reversals in readings, so I go by positions and the other cards. This card in this position tells me that her vital force was already ebbing: the tide was going out. This should have been the time in her life when she stopped all magical action and spent some years learning, resting, reflecting, and doing physical work

## 6. Tarot as a healing tool: interpretation

to rebalance the powerful magical work she had already accomplished. The fact that she stopped writing soon after this time is possibly an indicator that she was outwardly struggling. Magical writing in a contacted way takes a lot of energy and effort; something she had dwindling supplies of.

My conclusion, based on what I have seen in these readings, is that a train-wreck was already lining up a decade before her death. The choices we make during these key turning points decide if we are still going to be in a train-wreck, or if we are going to be able to avoid the collision—or at least survive it. She chose to continue on the path she was treading. I do not know if she was conscious of the fate that was before her, or if she knew about the path she had stepped onto. No one will ever know for sure.

From a purely magical health perspective, I then decided to look at her vital force at the point in time when she decided to do The Magical Battle of Britain work. Although she engaged people from all over the country to participate, and a massive, coordinated body of work was pulled together, she took the main magical burden of this working as she was its instigator on a magical level. This is a dynamic that a lot of people do not think about in terms of energy distribution and consequence: whoever holds the strings holds the burden of the Weaver. She was the holder of the strings, she coordinated, led, controlled the work, the method of work, the times, the dates, what her volunteers did, and how they did it. That level of control drops a massive burden on the back of the person who heads a major work in that way. So what state was she in when she took a hold of that bunch of strings? Let's have a look (fig. 6.4).

To get a straight simple answer to that question, we look at the last card. In the tenth position we find the Fool. The answer is that her vital force at the beginning of the Battle of Britain was almost non-existent. The number of the Fool is zero; the Fool with nothing steps off the cliff—and that was precisely what she did. Whether she did that in full knowledge as a sacrificial act, or whether she truly did not know what a fatal risk she was taking, we will never know.

It is easy to assume that an adept can 'see' everything: that is often not so, particularly when we come to ourselves. Seeing one's own future can be particularly hard at times, and easy at other times. I have had times of excellent clarity when I have foretold many things accurately within my own future. But

## 6.2. Diagnostic reading

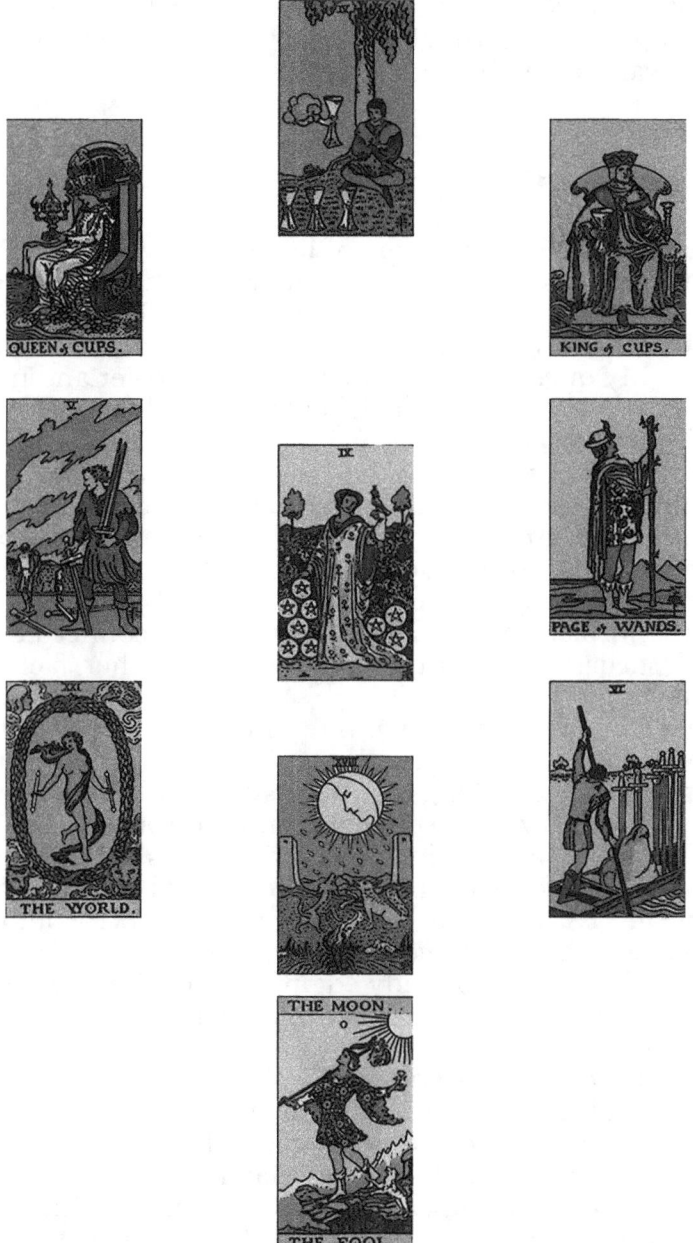

*Figure 6.4: Tree of Life reading: Dion Fortune's vital force at the beginning of the Battle of Britain.*

# 6. Tarot as a healing tool: interpretation

there have also been other times when seeing the future was like trying to see a car through the fog: you kind of see the lights, but you cannot get the details.

## 6.3 The last three years

To look at her last three years of life, which will show us what was going on for her at a deep level during the height of the Battle, I have chosen to use the Desert layout, which will indicate to us the magical dynamics flowing through her inner landscape (fig. 6.5). My question was: 'show me what power and magical dynamics were flowing through her Inner Landscape three years before she died.'

**The King of Pentacles** in the first position, which is the **body**, was something that stumped me. The King of Pentacles had shown up a few times in different readings about her, and usually showed as an inner contact. But this card is firmly positioned in her body. The only thing I can think of is that maybe a nature/land/faery/ancestral being could have connected to her magical sexual use of her mind. In other words, her 'faery lover' had moved in.

We tend to assume that parasites must be bad for our health, but sometimes a symbiotic relationship can develop that gives strength to the host along with access to knowledge that would not normally be available to them. If this person was alive today, I would do further readings to ask questions like 'is this card indicating another being living inside her?' 'Is that relationship beneficial?' 'Is that relationship harmful?' And I would most likely use a Tree of Life layout to get a straight answer. The other option is that she was already edging towards her ancestors by getting close to death: the King of Pentacles is also the king of ancestors.

The **three of swords** crossing her (in the **relationship** position) tells me that she was not in a direct relationship with any other human: she and Penry were divorced by this time, and it would seem from the details that have that she was not in a direct relationship with anyone else. It could also indicate her 'relationship' with her impending death: this is a pattern I have seen before in readings.

The **Queen of Wands** is in the 'stars,' i.e. the **long-term future**. This, along with the final card (these two positions are read together as long-term future and short-term future) tells

## 6.3. The last three years

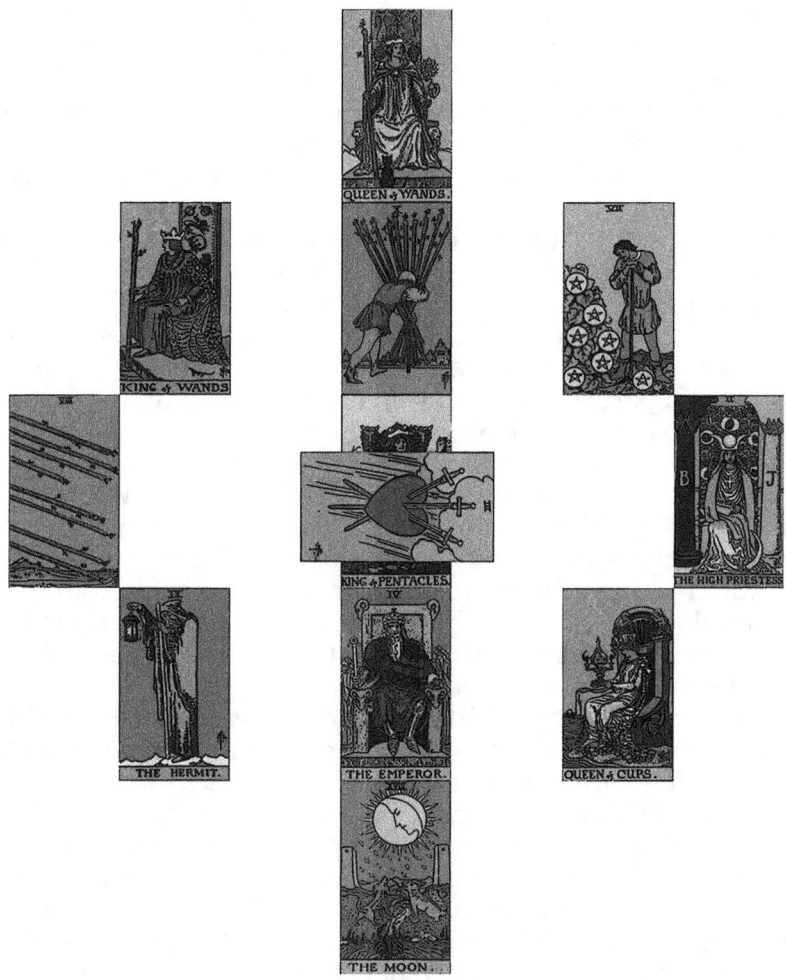

*Figure 6.5: Inner Landscape reading: 'Show me what power and magical dynamics were flowing through her Inner Landscape three years before she died.'*

## 6. Tarot as a healing tool: interpretation

me that although we know she was already on her last steps to death at this time, her long-term future was as a priestess.

Many would argue that she was already a priestess, which of course she was; but these two cards indicate that after her death she would step into a far more powerful octave of priestesshood. The Queen of Wands also indicates that she would move away from the qualities of the Queen of Cups, which was her indicator at this time of her life and a card she strongly identified with. She steps from magical West to magical South, into a pattern of fire magic. This could be as a priestess in another life, or as an inner contact.

In the **depths** is the **Moon**: the power of the moon, sea and water that she so strongly identified with. In this reading it has already passed, along with the veiled sight of a moon priestess: she was preparing to step into a very different power and role. This natural shift from the power of one magical direction to another is a part of our evolution as magicians and priest/esses, and this part of her life was the crossing of that threshold: her future was lining up, even as her death approached. This is something that I have seen repeatedly in readings with people who are quite close to their deaths: their next life or existence somehow begins its pattern before the old life is finished.

This crossing of thresholds that we see in DF's reading had profound implications for her deeper spirit, particularly in light of the ritual binding/banishing that was done to her after her death by some SIL folks.

In the position of the **immediate past** we have the **eight of wands**, which is mobile vitality/energy. Just as we saw in the Tree of Life reading, her vital force was already past.

In the position of **current patterns** is the **King of Wands**. Although she was not in a relationship with a man, she was definitely walking a fate path at this time with a male who was fiery and adventurous. To guess who would be simple speculation, but I would put my money on Crowley. Whoever it was, the fact that they show in her inner landscape pattern tells me that this male was a deep influence that crossed her path in order to help the transition from Queen of Cups to Queen of Wands.

In the position of the **mountain** is the **ten of wands**: burden. And it was indeed a Burden—with a capital B—that she was carrying. This is the weight of holding all the threads: coordinating everything at an inner and outer level for The

## 6.3. The last three years

Battle of Britain, keeping up her writing and teaching, as well as carrying the energetic burden of the fight for her country.

In the position of the Inner Temple, which tells us what is happening in regards to her inner work or inner contacts that work with her, is the card seven of pentacles. This is a 'good job!' card. So regardless of her energetic deficits, mistakes and emotive struggles, from an inner perspective she was indeed doing a good magical job, and that success was appreciated by the inner contacts/inner temples that she worked with.

In the position of **home/family** we have the **Queen of Cups**, which was the current way her 'family' i.e. the Society of the Inner Light saw her.

Falling away from her pattern and moving towards the **door of the past** we have the **Emperor**. Bearing in mind the context of the reading and the circumstances that surrounded her, I would take this to be Hitler on his way out. She was fighting to bring down the 'Emperor,' and that is precisely what happened.

In the position of **dreams/sleep/vision** is the **Hermit**. In the quiet of the night, and the depths of her dreams, in her meditations and visions, wisdom and introspection became her companion.

I do not doubt for a moment that this was the most profound time of her life for her and her alone. So much of her life was taken up being something for someone else; people wanted her to be Pagan, other people wanted her to be more Christian, people wanted her to be teacher, guide, boss, organizer, high priestess—but alone in the dark she faced herself in her depths. And what she saw was profound... and also disturbing.

This **culminates** eventually as the **Priestess**: as she stepped forward to her death, she also began to step into her true self. Whether that true self became another human life or an inner contact deep in the inner temples is irrelevant: what is important is that she made it.

If she was indeed parasited towards the end of her life (King of Pentacles), that would make a lot of sense as to why she behaved the way she did in the lodge/temple at the SIL after her death. She was eventually banished, and that action would have helped to tear away any 'hangers-on' and allowed her to move deeper towards her next pattern as the Queen of Fire.

We think in terms of lodges, hierarchies, grades and achievements. We think that this is the ladder of magic that we climb, and when we are older we will become great adepts.

## 6. Tarot as a healing tool: interpretation

Not true. Each life we live is a step on the ladder, a movement forward towards true magic.

### 6.4 General interpretation advice

You should now have a vague idea of how a magician can use tarot to look at health and magical effects on the body. One answer will often lead to more questions, and the layouts are chosen to gain the information that you need.

Always start with the heath layout, and make sure that you understand the basics of how the human body operates so that you can properly interpret what it is you are looking at. When you shuffle the cards, focus your mind on the question and make sure that the question you ask is clear. If you ask a question like, 'am I ill?' you are very likely to get a muddled reading. Things are always going wrong on some level with the body, and any imbalance will show up. That results in a busy and confused reading.

It is better to ask 'what effect did that magical work/action have on my general health?' If after a lot of magical work or a suspected attack you are finding that your body is not doing so well, or you are suddenly drained and not recovering, then a good question to ask would be, 'what is happening to my body?' If you suspect a magical impact or an attack, look to the first two cards of the reading: they will tell you if indeed there is a problem that is caused by magic.

If there is a benign card in position one but a volatile or difficult card in position two, then the problem could be magical or it could be a health condition that is just coming into form. In such circumstances it is useful to then use the Desert layout to check and see what is going on in your inner landscape.

If you still suspect an attack or a magical impact, then use the Four Directional layout to look at what elemental powers are flowing into your sphere. If you still suspect an attack, then ask a direct yes/no question using the Tree of Life: 'am I being magically attacked?' The final card, and the card in the eighth position, will give you your answer.

Read the elements in relation to the body: wands/fire for example can indicate infection, inflammation, aggression or a specific fire magic attack or impact. Too much of any element in the body can cause problems, so ensure that you understand the effects of elemental imbalance on physical heath.

## 6.4. General interpretation advice

The other and most important thing to bear in mind is not to frighten yourself. When you look close-up at a body situation and you get a lot of major problem cards show up, it could mean there is a major problem—or it can mean that it will *feel* like there is a major problem but really it is not too bad and it will pass. If you do get what potentially looks like a problem reading, then extend the timeline to look at the body over six or twelve months so that it can be put in context. When you get a good dose of the shits it can feel like you are going to die, or at least, you want to die! But it passes quickly and vanishes out of the reading within a couple of weeks.

Conversely, if a major destruction card repeatedly shows up in the same area, but you feel fine, do not ignore it. Explore further through readings to find out what caused it, what it is, and what it is going to do.

Many years ago I had the Tower repeatedly show up in the centre of my health reading. I felt fine, so I ignored it, as I did not understand it at the time. But in fact it was trying to show me a major illness that was developing as a result of a very nasty continuous magical attack that was still operating. The illness itself did not manifest for another two years, but if I had heeded the warning and looked properly, I could have dealt with it while it was still in its earliest stages. Sadly I did not, and the price I paid for that was repeated toxic medical treatments and surgeries.

I learned that hard lesson though, and now I watch my body like a hawk. Many people will sail through decades of magic with little effect besides the odd bump and scratch. If however you are like me and tend to explore, dig deeper, push boundaries—and incidentally piss off lots of emotionally infantile magicians who are nevertheless magically skilled, then you too will probably hit a major health issue at some point. The good side of that is that I learned a great deal during that time of ill-health, and I am still learning a lot about how amazing the human body is.

Keeping an eye on the body and caring for it is a major part of 'avoidance magic': that is to say, avoiding the major Towers that are unnecessary for your personal growth. You spot them and deal with them. By doing that you will learn a great deal about magical power, how it works, and how the strands of power can be woven so intricately. But on the other side of the coin there are certain Towers that cannot be avoided, and the initiatory illness is one of them (death is the other). What you can do is to learn how to live well despite them and to learn as much

## 6. Tarot as a healing tool: interpretation

as you can from them. Such necessary trials teach us patience, compassion, resilience, and stillness in the face of the whirlwind.

Chapter Seven

# *Visionary healing: part one*

## 7.1 Going down the rabbit hole

The use of visionary methods to aid the body in the healing and cleansing process is an important skill for the magician to learn. Any human can use the mind in order to trigger a healing or cleansing response, and this action engages the consciousness in an active conversation with the body. However, when such work is done by a magician who is trained or skilled in visionary magic, something very special happens: the consciousness becomes an active participant in an action that goes beyond the individual— it initiates a conversation not only with the body, but with the spiritual beings that flow all around us in the constant universal dance of creation and destruction.

This is one of the hallmarks of visionary work: engaging the conscious mind in a focused way to enable an action or reaction to occur within both the body and the spirit, in union with the many beings that are 'outside' of us.

This working in tandem with inner world beings is what separates visionary work from our own psychology. Psychological therapy uses visionary work or pathworking to achieve a deeper engagement with ourselves. Visionary magic uses visionary work in order to engage with inner beings and realms that are not our own, and which exist independently of us.

When a magician uses such techniques, and works within a magical healing framework or structure, two things happen: firstly, beings that are able to assist us are called upon, and secondly, the magician learns to partially dissociate themselves from their body in order to objectively 'treat' it. Our bodies are our vehicles; they are not our sole identity.

By learning how to work with the body in a team sense as opposed to a 'self' sense, the mind is able to engage healing and regenerative responses without the magician identifying themselves with the process. This is a very important step.

## 7. Visionary healing: part one

When the body becomes sick from a magical impact, attack or infestation, it is important not to take it personally or to personally identify with the problem. Such isolation pulls the magician away from the more toxic side of psychology that we have developed, and enables the magician to see clearly and without emotion.

Psychology has brought many wonderful things to our door, but it has also brought along many disabling elements, too. Rudolf Steiner began to understand the self's separate existence from the body, and to understand that we stand in line with many other beings that have no physical form, but which nevertheless affect our physical world. Unfortunately the world of science was unable or unready to accept such a concept, and Steiner's experiences were watered down and reinterpreted both by himself and his students in order to protect the awakening science of anthroposophy. But many magicians will look at his paintings, read his words, and nod with recognition at what this talented man was seeing as he peered behind the veil.

If you only reach within yourself for healing, knowledge and wisdom, you will pull from a very limited pot, while many inner beings stand around and observe you with amusement. If however you understand, particularly as a magician, that the world does not begin and end with you, that you are not god, that you are not all beings, and that you do not have a secret stash of wisdom consciousness hidden away in your armpit or somewhere that you could tap into if only you used the right psychology, then such an awakening of understanding will open your eyes to the true vastness of the consciousness that is all around us. We are a very small and insignificant part of the universe, and if we approach the universe properly, we can learn much, gain help and guidance, and become a part of the huge team called creation.

This understanding allows us to surrender our sense of control over everything and ask for help. Through divination, meditation and visionary work we can stand back, ask for advice, and look at the best way forward when we stand at a crossroads. The ability to open our eyes and 'see' is one of the most powerful gifts a magician can have. Magic is not about control; it is about informed choices.

With visionary healing, we engage that power of choice and reach out to the beings all around us to ask for assistance—and of course, we also offer that assistance back when it is needed. It is always a two-way conversation.

## 7.2 When to use visionary healing

In this day and age, we are programmed to think in terms of multiple choice questions, and we have a very black-or-white view on most things that we encounter. Life is really not like that, and there are no hard and fast rules as to when visionary healing is the appropriate healing method; often healing the body, soul and mind requires a complex pattern of different healing modalities, selected according to the flow of power both around and within the magician.

This is where divination comes in handy: it is important to work with your body in the way it needs at that specific time. Often those needs will either fluctuate unpredictably or ebb and flow predictably, so it is important to be pliable enough in how you approach your own healing in order to respond appropriately.

So for example, if a magician has taken a major impact or two which has damaged them, or they have become chronically ill, then it is likely that the healing process will include visionary work, herbs, homeopathy, acupuncture, allopathic medicine and rest—though not all at the same time!

The body is a very finely-tuned instrument, and becoming aware of its needs, its language and its energy fluctuations is important so that you can respond and change your healing approach as and when the body asks for it. Do not feel that you can just choose one healing method and run with it, and that such action would suffice; such an attitude is folly, and is a product of our modern 'go to' world. You cannot pop a pill or herb or do a vision and think everything will now be OK; healing is an unfolding process.

Visionary healing is often needed when there has been a major hit on the body, and the emotions, personality or mind have begun to show changes. It is also useful when there is or has been an infestation or a major disease that has an inner being behind it. The visionary work can run concurrent with proper medical care; the inner doctor and the outer doctor! Visionary healing can be overused and can hamper a person's recovery if it is used obsessively, but used properly it can massively speed up the healing process.

The keys to success are as follows: Look through divination: 'will this help the body?' Work with the appropriate visionary structure, and then let it do its work. If you are not cured after six hours, do not be tempted to try again! Visionary work done

## 7. Visionary healing: part one

on the body takes time to do its work. Sometimes you do feel a massive difference within twenty-four hours; sometimes it needs to bring on a healing crisis.

The methods of visionary healing work from the outside in: first you focus on the structure of the body (i.e. its organs, bones etc.). From there you step deeper in, and work with the energetic wheels that uphold the endocrine system. Then you move in still deeper to the subtle body and work with the flows of inner power, before finally working upon the inner pattern of manifestation itself that allows you to exist in the physical realm.

Always start from the outside in. Never go straight to the source pattern: to do so can sometimes shock the system. I used to work from the deepest point and then work outwards, but I found that doing so caused an unhelpful overreaction in the body. Working from the outside in allows the deeper energetic body to slowly adjust to the work, thus enabling a steady, stable response.

### 7.3  Stillness

In all of my books I rattle on about the need to learn how to be within stillness. I am that 'nagging aunt' for a very good reason: without stillness there *is* no visionary work. When you are sick or infested, it is hard to maintain stillness, but it is very important to do a stillness meditation every day, even if only for a few minutes. This also prepares you for visionary work, and allows you to focus on the job at hand. It also gives your mind and body space to begin the cleanup that it needs.

### 7.4  Cleaning and vacuuming, sewing and patching

A lot of visionary healing is very practical in its approach: you imagine the use of tools that you are familiar with in everyday life. If you see yourself cleaning the body out with a vacuum cleaner, you are signalling to an inner being working with you that you are trying to 'clean' the body.

Often modern spiritual healing methods engage abstract concepts that we do not fully understand, therefore any being trying assist us has no clue what it is we are trying to do. Use your conscious imagination as a vocabulary of communication:

## 7.4. Cleaning and vacuuming, sewing and patching

if you want to wash something, see yourself with a wet cloth and soap! It is that simple.

Often when the body is impacted from magic, or you have travelled in vision to an unhealthy place, there is a good chance that you are covered in spiritual dirt, gribblies (a highly-technical term for low-level parasitical beings!) etc. You may have been injured, torn something, or had a piece bitten out of you. In such cases visionary magic would be the first port of call, after which it would be wise to use herbs to mop up the residue and trigger healing.

This method can also be used when you have gone into a very bad place in the outer world, and have taken an energetic impact as a result. If the impact is big enough, a ritual cleansing bath will not be enough: you will also need to do an internal visionary cleaning. So how do you do it? Quite simply, really.

Light a candle, and do a stillness meditation. After a few minutes, call upon the deity you work with, or upon Divinity and the angelic beings that work between Divinity and humanity, or upon the Goddess within the land to guide and protect you as you work. This is an important step, as it immediately signals an intention to work with Divine forces which in turn alters the energetic frequency around you: this keeps you safe while you work. Note: do not call upon specific named angels—simply ask 'The Angels of Divinity' or 'Angels of the Lord' to assist you. This allows the appropriate angel to step in, the one who is best suited for the job.

There is no need for impressive rituals and callings. As a magician, simply stating your submission to the Divine force is enough to engage it at a passive level. If, however, you are working on something far more powerful than dirt and gribblies, then you will need a more targeted approach.

Close your eyes, and see the room around you in your mind. Step out of your body and stand before it in vision. Call upon the Father and the Mother to guide and watch over you as you work. See a tool kit and cleaning kit at the side of your body.

As you begin to work, you may become aware of beings working with you, handing you tools and taking the dirt away. It is also good to note that what you see as a vacuum cleaner is actually a being you are working with—the vacuum imagery simply enables you to work quickly and allows the being to get on with its job.

Look into the body to see any dark areas, small beings clinging onto the spine or neck, or around the pelvic region

## 7. Visionary healing: part one

or genitals. Look for grubs, eggs, and anything that looks like it should not belong there, and start to take them out using a vacuum cleaner. Vacuum throughout the body, making sure you get into all the corners, and pay particular attention to the spine and the brain.

When you are done with the vacuum, then get out the hosepipe and flush the body clean. If you see rips or tears in or around the body, sew or glue them back up. When you have finished cleaning the body, see yourself digging a hole in the floor down into the earth, and empty the vacuum bag into the land where it will compost. Once finished, come out of vision and immediately take a ritual salt bath, the method for which is outlined in the appendix.

This is the first stage of visionary healing, and it is the method used to clear the decks of low-level dirt and beings so that you can begin to work on what is *underneath* all that dirt, and to also begin to work on the body itself. This method of work is very 'shamanic' in its application; such an approach works well with the body, and there is no need for anything more ritualized or spiritualized. It is a matter of rolling your sleeves up and getting on with it.

### 7.5 The guardians of the organs

As you will have noticed, visionary healing starts from the outside and works in. Rather than going straight into deep spirit and working with the life force, it is better to start at the surface by cleaning up the body, ensuring that its physical substance is worked on before moving deeper into the more powerful thresholds within the body.

The reason for working from outside to inside, from mundane to spirit, is because such a graded process allows the body to adjust energetically at every step, and it therefore does not shock or burden the body. In today's world, we often think that more and stronger is better, which is not always the case, particularly where the body is concerned. The human body often responds far better to subtle hints than it does to shouting.

After the body has been cleaned, it is time to talk to the Guardians. You can talk to your own or you can talk to someone else's: like all of this work, it is both for personal use and for use in service to fellow magicians. Working with the Guardians of the Organs essentially means talking to the organs and to the spirits that reside within them.

## 7.5. The guardians of the organs

This is an alien concept to us in the West, and I fell across it while reading texts about acupuncture. When it comes to an unfamiliar magical technique, I first work with it practically to see if it does work, and then if it does, I explore further to see how it works, why it works, etc. And I can tell you, boy does this one work! It is also very interesting, and what it revealed certainly changed how I viewed my body. Who said you cannot teach an old dog new tricks...

Using visionary focus, sit quietly and meditate for a little while to settle everything down and become still. Once you are nice and quiet, be aware of yourself and of your body, and be aware of where your organs are and what they do. Focus first on the organ you feel is under the most stress, and using the same technique as 'cleaning your body,' go into your body in vision and look at the organ. Imagine the organ as a person, or a chamber with a person in it. This focused imagination creates an interface which allows you to interact with the spirit guardian or consciousness housed within the organ.

Look at what state they are in. Are they tired? Do they look ill? Do their surroundings look dusty or damaged? Talk to the guardian and tell them that you want to help. Clean up their area, wash them, and visualize them as full of power, well-dressed, and with a light or sunlight streaming into their space.

Work instinctively. When I worked with my heart, he looked like a tired old king in a dusty hall. I cleaned up the hall and imagined sunlight reaching him. As I was working, I got the strong impression that there were channels running around him that should be filled with water, but which were dry. I imagined the channels filling with fluid and flowing all around him.

Suddenly the old king woke up, and began to shine and look very regal. (And I felt the positive effect from that vision within an hour of finishing it.) I talked with him and checked that he was happy before I moved on to another organ.

Rather than look up any organ's attributes in the Five Spirit texts on acupuncture, I simply allowed the spirits to present themselves. By imagining a human interface, it lets the spirit interact with you and use your mind to create a common language. I did find, after I went back to the texts, that what I had 'imagined' corresponded pretty closely with what had been written. This is always the best way to work – find out for yourself what is there, and then check your observations with the textbooks.

# 7. Visionary healing: part one

After a few months of working this way and once communication was established, if a particular organ was struggling, it would 'tell' me: I would become very aware of the organ in question while going about my everyday life, and when that 'alarm' awareness happened, I would go in vision as soon as possible and talk to it. Often it needed some help or interaction.

This might all sound very strange, but hey—magic *is* strange, and it is important in magic to explore and find things out for yourself, rather than either dismissing a claim out of hand, or taking it on board without direct, personal experience.

I was quite astonished at the simplicity but also the effectiveness of this technique, but when I sat and thought about it, it did occur to me that we are, in fact, made up of many different beings. The human body houses masses of different bacteria, viruses, fungi, and God knows what else: we are a collective, and between us all we keep the body going. So it pays to know who your close neighbours are!

## 7.6  Colouring with the organs

This is closely connected with the concept of talking with the organs, but this particular technique looks at the energy around and within the organ. Essentially, the energy fluctuations of a body part can be perceived by visionary magicians in terms of colour. The identification of an energy by its colour is an old technique and one that has been long used in magic, but many magicians think of it as an intellectual attribute rather than a literal 'colour.' Nothing could be further from the truth. All energy vibrates at a particular frequency, and our brains can translate that frequency into colour or sound.

If an organ appears to have a red glow around it, then the chances are it is infected or inflamed. If it is grey, then it is probably lacking in energy and is breaking down. If the kidneys and adrenals are under stress, they too may appear red: allow your instincts to kick in when interpreting the colours rather than using any intellectual form.

If the organ is displaying a colour that is not right, simply imagine washing it with a colour that is healthier, calmer and more vital. When you have finished with the vital organs, imagine your body with all these different colours flowing in and around it. If you can, go and have a sleep after doing this work, so that the power can integrate properly and the organs can begin their regeneration processes.

If you practice this technique, you will find that it is very handy when you are suddenly under stress or fall ill; you can immediately direct the right frequency of energy to a particular organ to assist it in its rebalancing process.

## 7.7 Working with the endocrine system

This part of the human body can really take a hit from various forms of visionary and ritual magic if the work is prolonged and powerful. One of the various ways of healing such an impact is to work in vision directly with the glands themselves. Unlike the organs, the endocrine glands do not seem to have 'spirit guardians' so much as a dynamic that in Eastern meditation is known as the chakras. 'Chakra' means 'vortex' or 'wheel,' and that is exactly what appears in vision over the major glands. These wheels can be worked with and strengthened if the magician has good visionary skills.

A word of caution: if you are using this work on someone else to assist in their healing, and if they are very sensitive, be careful not to overstimulate these power glands. I once inadvertently overstimulated a thyroid gland in a sensitive visionary by being too enthusiastic in the work I did on them.

The magician was suffering from an impacted thyroid which had become very slow. I stimulated the gland, and twenty-four hours later I had a frantic magician at my door who was whizzing around like a hummingbird—oops. So tread carefully. You can always do a bit more work on a gland if it doesn't respond, and it is easier to give a gland more impetus than it is to slow it back down again if you overstimulate it.

The wheels work down the body from above the head to the groin, and then finally down to the earth. The first wheel, which appears over the top of a person's head, is in magical terms an energetic anchor that filters that person's future. The second wheel appears at the forehead, and stimulates the hypothalamus, pineal and pituitary glands. These three glands work in tandem, and the pineal in particular is more active in visionary magicians than in the ordinary person in the street. The pineal seems to work as a primal anchor, with the hypothalamus and pituitary busying themselves with keeping stasis and filtering power.

The next gland to have a wheel over it is the thyroid, and then below that the thymus. Just under the sternum is the pancreas which also has a wheel, and in the position of the umbilicus is the wheel that affects the adrenals. The groin also has a wheel which

## 7. Visionary healing: part one

governs the sexual organs, and the final wheel, which often does not appear on Eastern medicine charts, is the grounding wheel which appears just under the feet.

These wheels chart a line through the body and beyond, and linked together they form a power highway axis that the rest of the body operates around. They work in tandem, and should all be running at the same speed. When working in vision with these wheels, if you find one that is not running at the same speed as the others, it identifies a problem in that area of the body.

To work in vision with these wheels, lie down and still yourself. When you are sure you are still, visualize yourself within the body and be aware of these wheels. To some they appear within the body, but for me they always appear just above its surface, hovering over my skin.

I have developed a visionary language so that I can interface with these wheels, and that visionary language is to see them as mechanical wheels with cogs at their base and a setting indicator at the top. The indicator dial has twelve settings, with the sixth setting at twelve o'clock: this is the default setting that they should all run at to be healthy.

The wheels all have their own unique energetic 'light' and colour, which seems to vary from person to person. Using your imagination, start with the wheel above your head, and build an awareness of its brightness and setting. If it is dark, it will need cleaning and light bringing into it to energize it. I imagine a well of energy at my umbilicus that I can draw from to brighten up dull wheels.

When I have worked on these wheels both on myself and other people, I did notice that the first and last (over the head and under the feet) had no setting range, just brightness and colour. So start from the top wheel and work on its colour and brightness. As you work to energize it, you will instinctively become aware if its colour is not right: trust your instinct and experiment—it is the best way to learn!

When you move down to the wheels that are over the glands, you will become aware of their settings, cogs, base, etc. If the setting is too low or too high, adjust it (I see myself turning a knob until the pointer is at midpoint). If it will not move, it may have a blockage. If that is the case, then imagine getting into the cog underneath the wheel where it 'plugs' into the body, and see if there is any stuff blocking it.

## 7.8. The inner landscape

I say stuff, because when I see it, it is like dirty glue or a calcified build-up. I just clean it off, grease the mechanism down, and set it off again. Work with the imagination in ways that are familiar to you: imagine cleaning cogs and wheels, washing things down, brushing them, and if the energy is low, imagine a hosepipe from the stars that runs to your energy pot in your umbilicus to 'fill the tank' back up. By using such familiar images, your body, spirit, and any other beings around you know what it is you are trying to do.

Work your way down the body, take note of ones going too slow or too fast, reset them and finish with the energetic one under your feet. If one is going slow and refuses to speed up, then it is probably going slow for a reason. If there is infection or something invasive going on in that region of the body, the wheel that sits over or close to it will slow down as the body tries to fight whatever it is fighting. I am guessing here, but chances are it is slowing down to stop any invader having access to the energy it dispenses.

A few times when I have worked on people, one of their wheels would just not budge its speed even after it had been cleaned and energized. Without fail, a few days later that person would get sick, and the sickness would focus on the area near the slowed wheel. After their immune system had done its job and suppressed the invaders, the wheel would speed up again. I found that absolutely fascinating.

To me (and I may be stating something that everyone except me already knew) it would seem that these wheels are like an energy highway for the body. Just as the endocrine glands function as controllers, communicators and governors, the 'inner' endocrine system—these wheels—distribute energy to those glands and their surrounding organs in order to help them work.

If when you are working on these wheels you find that one of them is out of rhythm, use the method of going into the body in vision, and look around the affected area: look at the organs, nerves and bones, and see if you can find where the problem lies.

## 7.8 The inner landscape

This technique is an interesting and powerful way to look at the overall health of a body, to spot disturbances at a deep psychic level, to see if there are any unwelcome spirits deeply embedded

## 7. Visionary healing: part one

within the container of the body, and to look at the deeper personality or the soul of the person.

To access the inner landscape I use a simple visionary interface: I use vision to go into the body, up the spine and into the brain. I move deep into the centre of the brain, and there I 'see' a doorway. I go through the doorway, and up some old stone steps which open out onto a landscape.

When I first came across this level of the body's consciousness, I worked within people's landscapes to initiate healing; but I gradually found that making changes in this place seemed to shortcut their long-term, deep soul learning. I learned eventually not to tinker with a person's inner landscape, but to merely observe and take note: it would give me a great deal of detail about how deep the damage was, and that information would then guide me as to what sort of healing was necessary.

The inner landscape does not appear as an inner body; rather it appears as a nature landscape. For years I could not understand why it should appear this way, but the deeper I delved into visionary Kabbalah, the more it made sense. The landscape is Malkuth: the container of the Divine Spark, the manifest world, and everything that physically appears in the physical realm. Every physical thing that manifests is a container for Divinity, and the first expression of that manifestation is the land. The living beings all sprang from the landscape—we truly are children of the Great Mother.

When you look at a person's inner landscape, take note of the weather, of the land itself, the nature that is alive (trees, plants, water, rock) and any beings that are present besides the person themselves. Most people appear in their landscapes, and how they appear will tell you a great deal about the state of their deeper spirit.

Do they appear as children? Do they appear old or young, healthy or ill, strong or faint? What type of landscape do they have? Is it barren, fruitful, balanced with land and water; is it a garden, is it in a state of nature, or is it a harsh and lifeless landscape?

I found over the years that bad weather such as storms would herald illness or infection, a lacklustre landscape indicated low energy, and a lack of landscape or a chaotic one would often indicate more serious mental issues. I have come across landscapes that do not have any nature within them at all, and I eventually learned that such people seemed 'new' to humanity, as if they did not understand nature or humanity at all; it is

## 7.8. The inner landscape

as if they came from some other realm that had little or no connection with humanity.

Occasionally I came across other beings in a landscape, and I learned that often they were trying to move into a person and establish themselves. Often a sharp telling-off and showing them 'the door' would get rid of them, but by doing this I bypassed the person's own inner immune system, and they did not learn how to defend themselves from such an invasion. I eventually figured out that it is better to work at a more 'surface' level with the endocrine system, organs, brain, and nervous system, followed by ritual bathing, so that the body itself expelled the intruder.

I also found, mainly in more vulnerable teens and young adults, that occasionally when a person was in an abusive relationship, their abuser would appear in their landscape, as if they had bypassed the natural boundaries of the spirit and were operating energetically at a deep level in the victim's psyche. Obviously this is not intentional on the abuser's part, but that type of person seems to have a natural ability literally to 'invade' someone. In such cases I simply took note and worked at more outer levels to strengthen the person emotionally, so that they could eventually break the connection for themselves. That way, their own inner immune system could learn and mature.

If you are working within your own landscape it is a slightly different situation. There are times when it is okay to work on your own landscape, and there are times to simply observe, take note, and act from an outer approach. If you do find a being wandering about your inner landscape, simply tell it to fuck off out (ancient ritual words!) and then work from a more outer perspective to strengthen your mind, body and energy so that it cannot happen again.

As with all deeper magic, there are no hard and fast lists of rules to follow. You must learn the basics first, and then work instinctively, use divination to track your progress and options, and learn by practical experience. The more you work, the more you will learn for yourself and discover your own vocabulary of practice.

Every culture around the world has its own versions of this type of work in their mystical texts; the key is to not be dogmatic but to understand that they are talking from their own time and culture, and that none of us have all the answers. It is better to use texts as signposts but walk the path yourself, and adjust your work according to what you find, how it works, and what reactions you have to it.

# 7. Visionary healing: part one

## 7.9 Working with the patterns of life force

This is the deepest form of visionary healing that can be done on a person, and it works at the threshold where the spirit and the body come together to exist as a living human. This level of visionary healing works with the power of the weaver: a pattern within the Mysteries that presents itself in the inner desert at the edge of the Abyss in the form of a web of geometric patterns made up of angelic beings.

Those beings create thresholds and filters for the Utterance of Divinity to flow through into manifestation. Everything in creation has octaves, and the web pattern found deep in the inner worlds as a filter for manifestation also presents at a lower octave in our bodies. We too have a threshold pattern that allows the Utterance of Divinity to flow into us, giving us our life force. Sometimes, that web can get damaged and needs attending to.

In the ordinary everyday person, such a breakdown of the pattern is connected with ageing and long-term disease: it is a part of the destruction process that will eventually lead someone to their death. In a magician, such damage to the pattern can also come about from magical impact, attack, or a power issue. In these cases it is important to repair the damage at the deepest level.

If a magical impact or attack damages the pattern at this level, no matter what other healing is done, the magician will neither fully recover nor have their power restored if their pattern of life is torn. The best way to tell if the magician is damaged at this level is to look via readings.

To work at this level of healing it is useful to plug into something more powerful than yourself. Whereas all the other healing methods rely on the magician and the usual beings around him or her, working with the pattern of life is far more effective if the magician plugs themselves into the deeper pattern at the edge of Abyss. This involves working in two places at once and bringing the octaves together. It requires a good working knowledge of the Kabbalistic inner desert, a familiarity with working at the edge of the Abyss with the pattern of manifestation, and the ability to work with angelic beings in vision.

The first step of this work is to go in vision into the inner desert and walk to the edge of the Abyss. Turn around to face down the desert/Tree of Life with the intention of working with

## 7.9. Working with the patterns of life force

the pattern of manifestation. This pattern appears at the edge of the Abyss and is akin to watching angelic beings play cats cradle.

Walk through the pattern (doing this triggers your own pattern), and continue walking within the pattern as you move down the desert/tree and step over the threshold of Malkuth.

See yourself walking into mist with the intention of going to your own body or the body you will be working on. Also be aware of angelic beings walking behind you as you emerge out of the mist. You do not need to communicate or interact with them; rather your approach and intention tells them what you are about to do.

As you walk out of the mist, the building where your body is emerges in front of you: step into the building, go to the body, and look at it. Give yourself time to adjust as you look into the body: have the intention of seeing the web pattern of manifestation in the body—it usually fans out from the umbilicus in all directions. Look for breaks in the pattern, frayed bits, or signs of tearing or impact. One of the angelic beings will position themselves behind you and will work through you, their arms through your arms.

Don't allow your intellect to intervene; it is better to work instinctively so that the beings behind you can work properly through you. Let your hands work like a spider, reweaving and reattaching, with threads coming out of your hands as you weave. Make sure that all the threads coming out of the umbilicus are reattached to where they should be, and that all the lines that were broken are rewoven. Once you have finished, it is then time to ensure that life energy can run properly through the pattern.

Look at the point from which all the threads originate, the point of the umbilicus. If you look closely, you will see that they seem to emerge from a small well. Make sure the well is clear of blockage so that power can flow properly.

There are two actions that can be done now to ensure the strength of life flows properly through the person. The first is to energize the pattern itself, to fill it with life force. Reach down into the tiny well at the umbilicus until you feel the life force, and pull it up to the surface. The pattern should immediately light up and glow brightly. This will also show you if there are any hidden tears that you missed.

The second action is to strengthen the person's spirit so that they are properly seated in their energetic and physical body. To do this, go behind the body and look at the back of the neck.

# 7. Visionary healing: part one

An angelic being will understand what it is you are about to do and will stand behind you. As you look at the base of the neck, you will notice a small opening that looks a little like a mouth: place your lips just in front of the mouth and you will feel the angel doing the same behind you. The mouth on the back of the neck of the body will react to your presence and will open slightly.

A noise will build up behind you, like muttering and singing. You will feel the angelic being placing their mouth on the back of your neck and breathing: this will cause an immediate build-up of power within you, a power that vibrates like a lot of voices. Open your mouth and let that power/vibration flow through your neck and out through your mouth: it will flow straight into the neck and body that you are working on.

The power pattern of the body will begin to vibrate and produce its own sound, and the sound that has flowed through you will join in. It becomes a symphony of life: all life is a vibration or frequency of power, and this action refocuses, reaffirms and reawakens the deepest part of a person, reminding them who they are. This action is a much lower octave of the Divine action of uttering a being into life, what is known in the Bible as 'The Word.'

This magical action is a profound and difficult one, which will leave you tired. It is important to sleep after doing this work, regardless of whether you do it on yourself or on someone else. It is not to be done lightly, and must only be done when absolutely necessary.

## 7.10 Summary

Visionary magic that focuses specifically on working directly with the body and within the body can be a powerful tool in the healing process. It gives the healing process a strong energetic foundation that the outer healing can stand upon: no matter what concoctions you give a person, if they have low vital force or are damaged at an inner level, the healing will not be successful or sustained until the deeper healing is done.

The methods of visionary healing that we looked at in this chapter work directly between magician and body. Sometimes we need a little more help if we have been knocked heavily, or the healing work needs to be done in a more structured visionary form. This is when the magician goes in vision to various realms to work with beings or deities who will intervene and assist in the healing process. That is what we will discuss in the next chapter.

Chapter Eight

# *Visionary healing: part two*

## 8.1 The call for help

Sometimes a magician can get so battered down from working powerfully in magical service that they need a helping hand from the inner worlds. A major impact cannot be fixed by doing a single vision, but working carefully with a deity both in vision and through protection magic over a period of time can assist dramatically with the healing process.

If the magical impact has caused chronic infection or a sustained immune response, then it is best to work with underworld deities and visions in order to help the body fight the infection. If the inner pattern of the magician has been damaged, then one method of approaching that problem is to work with angelic beings and the patterns of life itself while in vision. None of these methods are a replacement for wise actions, medicine, and caring correctly for the body, but they are among many of the tools that an experienced magician can use to help repair and regenerate it.

If you are planning to work with a deity in vision for deep healing, then it is a good idea to know what power you are working with, and whether it is the right power for what you are trying to achieve. Most of the deities that work well in this type of visionary healing are the ancient and underworld goddesses: they are vessels who hold both regeneration and destruction within their power. The older and more stable the goddess, the more successful the work will be.

I work a lot with Sekhmet, who is a goddess of both destruction and regeneration (her most regenerative healing aspect also appears as Hathor). She poisons and spills epidemics out into the world, but she also carries the cures for such calamities: every powerful deity will have both sides of a power dynamic within their repertoire.

If a magician has been working deep in the underworld or the Abyss, or has been attacked by beings or forces that are

## 8. Visionary healing: part two

generated in these places, then the most likely presentation of illness from such contact will be an infection of the mind or body. In such a case it is to the underworld that we turn to for help: always work with powers that are familiar with the issue.

In this chapter we will look at a specific visionary pattern for Sekhmet, before going into broader, less-defined areas of visionary healing. The vision that works with Sekhmet will show you how the structure works when you approach a powerful deity for healing. The other forms of visionary healing in this chapter have a broader sweep that the magician can adjust as needed for their own personal work.

### 8.2 Working with Sekhmet

Why Sekhmet? Most magic we encounter in the Western world has deep roots in the land of Egypt and the surrounding areas of Mediterranean North Africa, the Near East, and Southern Europe. Sekhmet is a very old deity and a form of the Underworld Goddess who appears within the land throughout Europe, North Africa, and the Near and Middle East. Neolithic portrayals of her have been found in Europe, and she is a power who presents herself often in deep magical work.

Her Egyptian form as Sekhmet is an interface that has been used for millennia, and her temple images still stand *in situ*— this is very important when reaching for an ancient deity: if the outer magical and ritual structure is still there, it is much easier to tap into the contact.

If you wish to work with her, it is wise to have good manners as she is a powerful and fierce goddess (alternatively you can work with Hathor; go where your instinct tells you to go). Having an image of her at home or in your temple where you can sit and talk with her, work with her, and give her offerings (a lit candle, a bowl of water etc.) will create a good working relationship. It is not about worship but respect, and honouring a power that is far greater than you are.

By first building a relationship with Sekhmet in such a way, it not only makes it easier to work with her in depth in vision, but it also gives you brownie points: she is more likely to be willing to help you if you honour her properly.

To approach her in vision in her Underworld temple (as opposed to visiting her in a surface-world temple) is to meet her at her most powerful. Be aware that nothing can be hidden from her, and a deep undercurrent of Ma'at runs through her:

## 8.3. Vision of Sekhmet

she is the defender of Ma'at, and of the order of life and death. If you approach her with selfishness, with hidden unbalanced intent, or to greedily ask for power, she will tear you apart. But if you approach her with openness, seeking her help after being damaged while acting in service, then she will become both Sekhmet and Hathor: the defender and the healer.

Because of the primal depths of Sekhmet's power and the strands of life that she holds, it is important that you place yourself before her at some point in your magical life, no matter how scary she can be. The vision of Sekhmet works on two different levels. The first level connects you to the formalized temple structure that has been built around her, and the second level of the vision takes you into direct contact with her power before it became too heavily formalized.

## 8.3 Vision of Sekhmet

For effective use, record this vision or have someone record it for you, and follow it passively for the first time or two. This enables you to learn the 'path' to Sekhmet. Once you know the way there, then it is important to be able to do the vision for yourself without recordings or help from others.

To prepare for the vision, have a candle lit before a traditional or ancient image of Sekhmet, and sit down quietly. Do not lie down, as it is important not to fall asleep during this vision. Close your eyes and go into the stillness. Meditate for a few minutes to totally still yourself and prepare for work.

With closed eyes, imagine that you can see the candle flame before you using your inner vision. As you look at the flame, remember your intent to visit the underworld temple of Sekhmet. As you think about that temple, a large hole opens up in the ground before you and the candle plunges down it, deep down into the land. You watch the candle fall, and decide to follow it. Jump into the hole. Do not fear it, or fear falling: trust, and jump.

Your body turns and tumbles as you fall deeper and deeper into the land, and the light of the surface world vanishes above you, leaving you to fall in darkness. You fall and fall, deeper and deeper into the land, entering the Underworld as you fall. You can hear water running around you, but you see nothing as you fall down and down. A wind comes up from beneath you, and seems to slow your falling until you almost come to a stop. You land in water, finding yourself surfacing and swimming

## 8. Visionary healing: part two

in an underground lake, but it is dark, and you can barely see anything. The only source of light is a flame in the distance, and you swim towards it.

The closer you get to the flame, the lighter the cavern becomes, and more flames appear. As you look around, you see that you are in a deep Underworld temple that is vast. The ceilings of the cavern are all painted deep blue with golden stars, and the closer you get to the lights, the more you notice large stone columns appearing on either side of you. The lights guide you to some rough-hewn steps that lead you out of the water and into the temple.

Climbing out of the water, you stand and look in awe at the vast ancient place in which you find yourself. Before you is a parade of colossal columns, all beautifully and colourfully decorated. The columns seem to go on forever and vanish into clouds of steam and smoke in the distance.

Something draws you to the smoke, which smells strongly of tree resins, and as you walk into the smoke you are bathed in the sacred perfume of temple incense in preparation for meeting the great Sekhmet. Something pushes you to move forward, and as you emerge out of the smoke you find yourself standing before a vast statue of Sekhmet that seems to be a hundred feet high. Between her colossal feet is a doorway, and in front of the doorway is a stone table or oblong altar.

Bow deeply to the ancient goddess and reach into your pocket. Whatever you find there, you offer to her.[1] As you place the offering before her, the doors between her feet open, and priests comes out. They indicate for you to get onto the altar, and to lie down. Once you lay down, they begin to work on your body by pulling things off of you, cleaning you, using medicines on your skin, and working energetically on you. Be still and let them work for however long it takes.

When they have finished, they step back and indicate for you to get off the altar and to enter the doorway between the feet of the goddess. As you step over the threshold of the door, you peer inside the chamber: it is dark, you can hear water dripping,

---

[1] If the object in your hand is something you own in your everyday life, then after the vision it must be given to her either by burying it, throwing it into a lake or river, giving it away to someone, or by burning it. It does not matter how valuable it is, you must give it to her. If it is something like your house keys, then be willing in your heart and mind to let it go. If you lose your house under such circumstances, then it is a good thing out of a bad—you no longer belong there and it is holding you back. It is important to learn to let go, to trust, and not to cling.

## 8.3. Vision of Sekhmet

and it smells strange. A hand pushes you from behind, and you stumble into the space as the doors slam shut behind you.

You find yourself in total darkness, but you can hear and smell a great deal. There is water all around you, and you can hear panting, like a large animal. A strong smell of lions fills the air, along with the smell of moss, damp stones, and earth. A light appears like a small oil lamp, and you gravitate towards it, treading carefully.

The lamp's flame slowly grows bigger so that you begin to see the cave in which you are standing. As you look around, you see a large, rough cave with many ancient primitive drawings painted on its walls. A small stream of water runs through the cavern, and the ground is littered with moss-covered rocks.

At the far end of the cave is a deep recess, and a fleeting movement in it catches your eye. Drawing closer you see an outline emerging, but it is not until you are very close that you see the two flashing lion eyes and the large outline: before you sits a tall black woman with the head and paws of a lion and the torso and limbs of a human. She is watching you to see how you will react to her. No matter how scared you are, inch closer and bow to honour her: this is Sekhmet in her true and most powerful form.

As you bow before her, she reaches out with a claw and scratches you deeply on the forehead. Blood runs down your face, and she moves closer to you to lick your face clean. The scratch has opened something in you, and you feel a deep shift in your body and mind. Sekhmet leans over you and breathes over the wound on your forehead, her breath reaching deep into your brain.

She sits back into the shadows as waves of darkness engulf you. You find yourself falling into darkness, tumbling around your memories and thoughts. The thoughts and memories slowly fade away as you fall through the darkness, until finally you stop falling and your mind moves into stillness and silence. There is no movement, no breath, no time, no thought: you drift in silence and your mind is calm, still and centred. This state fills you with peace and stability. Nothing intrudes, nothing demands; you simply *are*.

Within that stillness you slowly become aware of earth and rock all around you, of the roots of trees, the trickle of underground water, and the sleep of the ancestors who lie beside you. You are deep in the earth, at peace, in stillness—and yet you are still at the feet of the most ancient Lioness Goddess. A

# 8. Visionary healing: part two

noise distracts you from the stillness. Someone is calling your name.

Your mind follows the sound, the sound becomes a pattern, and the pattern becomes a web that you can traverse. You follow the path of the web which takes you from that deep, still place in which you were drifting to a place where you stand before a seated human.

It takes a moment for you to realize that you are standing before your own body. You see the threads of the web that stretches from your body and falls deep into the underworld: you are anchored in the presence of Sekhmet, and yet you are back in your own world before your own body. Step back into your body, and sit for a moment before opening your eyes: get used to the feel of being connected deep in the earth while still being conscious in your body. When you are ready, open your eyes, and meditate for a short while.

The deep vision of Sekhmet (which you should take your time with) is a long and difficult vision, but it connects you back to the ancient consciousness within the land, which in turn gives you an anchor that helps you to rebuild your strength. It also opens the gate within you to the most ancient goddesses within the land who hold this lioness power, a gate through which power, service and healing can run in both directions.

You must never place yourself at Sekhmet's feet if you are not willing to be aware of the Divine consciousness within the earth, and to offer service to the ancient powers that reside in the land. These powers will assist you if you are willing to be of service to the land, and to the Titan powers that run through it: one day you may be asked to work magically to support these deeper powers as they emerge within humanity, or to work with the elements to support the land in its recovery from the damage that humans have wrought.

## 8.4 Repairing the pattern

In the previous chapter, one of the magical acts of healing that we looked at was the action of repairing the inner pattern that allows you to manifest as a living being. Sometimes if a magician takes a big enough hit, the strain of working upon ones own pattern is too much of an energetic burden: if you are very low in energy but are still able to work in vision, then it is good to go and get some help.

## 8.4. Repairing the pattern

The safest place to have your inner pattern worked on while you are vulnerable is in a star temple which can be found hidden within the Inner Library. The Inner Library is a magical realm that is extremely stable, well guarded, and has endless branches connecting it to temples and priesthoods throughout time.

There is a part of the Inner Library that houses a fragment of the consciousness of arch-angelic beings that build, hold, and destroy the patterns of physical manifestation: they work to the rhythm of the Fates and the Weaver.

If you go in vision to the Inner Library with the express intent to work with these beings, you will be guided through the library's many different areas to the great circular door that is the threshold of these beings.

Once you step inside that chamber, you will be confronted by vast beings that seem to be holding complex patterns of threads in place, a bit like cat's cradle. Walk under the threads to the far side of the hall, and you will find slightly smaller angelic beings who will be able to help you. They will ask you to lie down while they stand over you and begin to reweave you, repair tears, etc.

You might well have to return to this place a few times to have the repairs done bit-by-bit. Follow your instincts, and do not waiver from your path to this chamber; do not get distracted in the Library. It is important to be focused and yet to surrender control over what is done to you in this place.

I had to use this method after I sustained a major magical impact when my energies were already low. I went in to the vision once every seven days for three weeks to have the repair-work done. After my first visit to this chamber, nothing much happened that I could notice: I did not seem to feel any different. But after the second and third visit, I noticed that I was starting to get an immune response: I got a really bad cold. I thought I must have been working in the wrong way, but the inner advice I was getting was to continue with the visions.

After the last visit, my cold resolved and I really started to feel good and strong. I ate like a horse and slept like the dead for a week, after which I emerged in full fighting form once more.

Something that we have lost touch with in this day and age of treating symptoms rather than the disease is that the body often needs to go through a healing crisis, where things are brought to a head and resolved. This is something that our forefathers understood very well, but it is a wisdom we have all but lost through our habit of seeking a drug that will instantly make us feel better, but which often just masks the disease by suppressing

## 8. Visionary healing: part two

the symptoms. For true healing, our bodies need to go through various stages of acute symptoms while the body gears itself up, followed by a phase of slower recuperation as the dust settles.

If after doing this work you have a similar reaction to mine, just go with the flow: let your body do what it needs to do, and support it without suppressing any of the shifts it is attempting to make. Once the body is on its way to the resolution phase of the healing process, then you can begin with herbs, rest, acupressure, etc. to support the healing without stopping the shifts that need to happen.

### 8.5 Finding the right realm and contacts for the job

Using vision to seek assistance is a major way of repairing underlying damage to the body and spirit, which then leaves the more surface manifestations to be dealt with using herbs and more body-based, externalized healing methods. A vast number of realms, deities, and inner contacts can be connected to for such healing, and which ones you should use largely depends on what land you live upon, what magical work you do, and what deities you are already connected to.

It is a good idea to seek help from within the circle of inner contacts and realms that you regularly work with. So, for example, if your magical work is very much geared towards faery and land-based magic, then that should be your starting-point. If you work as a Kabbalist, then the inner structures of the desert, inner temples, and angelic beings would be the place to begin. For the magician who works within a set tradition with deities, then looking for the appropriate deity within that tradition will bear good fruit. It is all about using your common sense.

However if you are an eclectic magician (as I am) and have moved beyond traditional paths, then you will probably find that one area of your practice will shout loudly for you to use that method or contact. Using divination to decide the right course of action goes without saying, and the level of power contact you decide to approach should be proportional to the level of damage you have sustained.

So, for example, curing a minor impact does not need a huge, powerful angel—an inner contact in the Library will be able to help with that. Conversely, a massive, life-threatening impact cannot be adequately handled by a local faery being.

Use your common sense, and if you are still not sure, turn the situation around in your mind and view it in terms of everyday life. Would you go to the local Reiki healer if you had a compound fracture? No, you would go to a hospital.

The one thing I will caution you about is to not use these methods to 'heal yourself' if what you are suffering from is simply a matter of you having a shit time in life, where 'no one loves you and the world is all against you.' If you have issues, stop looking in your navel, and sort your life out by direct engagement and action.

These powerful methods and contacts are not there to take your hand and baby you, or to deal with your own emotional and mental inadequacies. It is up to you to do everything in your power to sort yourself out and to get yourself back on your feet. You deal with your own personal dramas; the inner lot deal with energetic impacts that could potentially kill you or disable you.

## 8.6 Approaching a contact for healing

Once you have decided which deity or contact to approach for healing, you need to think carefully about what type of visionary interface to use in order to obtain the healing that you need. Rather than constructing a new interface, which takes a lot of time and energy which you most probably do not have, look to use an interface that is well-established.

Choose the interface (underworld, Inner Library, desert, faery realm, etc.) and before you do anything in vision, spend some time in a stillness meditation. From that stillness, pass into the visionary interface, and do not be distracted or allowed to be led into a different space: if you are weak, then you are vulnerable. If the interface you are working within has known guardians you can call upon, then do so.

Allow the deity or contact to work upon you, and when they have finished, leave a gift for them or agree to return the favour when called. Ensure that you stick to the bargain, and if you leave a gift in vision, ensure that whatever it was that you gave them is also given up in the material realm. So, for example, if you gave your favourite ring to the Goddess, then once you are out of vision you must get that ring and throw it in the nearest river. It does not matter how expensive it is: a gift is a gift.

When giving a gift, do not think about what you can get away with: if you hand opens and something of great value (financially

## 8. Visionary healing: part two

or emotionally) appears, do not even for a second think about changing it to something of less worth to you. Letting go is an important dynamic for magicians to learn, and there is also an interesting connection with what appears in your hand and what you need to learn to let go of.

After you have finished the vision, go and sleep. This is an essential part of visionary healing: the work continues in your body long after the vision has ended. By sleeping, you allow the powers to deepen within you.

## 8.7 Summary

Visionary healing is about dealing with energetic/magical injury and impact at the deepest level. On its own it is not a cure-all; but it will repair your foundations and reconnect your body and spirit back with your energetic resources so that your healing process can begin properly. Once you have worked on yourself in vision, give the body some time (i.e. a week or so) to absorb the experience before beginning more surface levels of treatment such as alternative medicine or even allopathic medicine.

Also be aware that deep magical impacts often have return resonances, whereby each year to the date of the original impact, the body experiences an echo of the event. You may get flare-ups of old injuries, dreams that put you back in the situation, or a lesser but similar event happening. Don't worry too much about this if it happens, as it is very common and perfectly normal. Just take note and see if there are any loose ends that need attending to. The echo will fade over time, but it may take two or three years to pass if the original event was a big one.

Chapter Nine

# *Homeopathy*

## 9.1 Little pills that pack a punch

Homeopathy is a fascinating form of treatment, particularly if you are a magical person. It is neither the panacea that it is often presented as, nor the sham that the drug companies and mainstream Western medical practitioners would have you believe it is. After twenty years of working with it, I now call homeopathy 'magic in a bottle,' because that is exactly what it is. Homeopathy is complex, and it can be very powerful or totally useless depending on how it is applied. These days it has been relegated to the corner of 'feel-good' medicine with a sprinkling of New Agey-ness thrown in; a form of treatment that people turn to when all else has failed.

In such cases it will usually not work. As a treatment for chronic disease, if there is poor vital force or the person lives a very toxic life, homeopathy will have little or no effect. Also, it can only rarely be applied as a one-size-fits-all treatment for illness: unlike an antibiotic, a homeopathic treatment is applied not to the illness but rather to the person. So while ten people on a hospital ward with the same illness can all be given the same drug in allopathic medicine, in homeopathy they would most likely all be given different substances at different strengths, depending on the person, their presentation of the illness, and so forth. So you can see how homeopathy can never really become a mainstream medicine: there are too many ill people, and not enough time.

With magicians it is different again. When you work in depth with magic, it changes how the body reacts to certain energies, including homeopathy; so often the basic rules of application change. This is why it is important to be able to work with the health layout covered earlier: you can look at the potential effects a remedy will have on you and choose the correct potency with full knowledge of what it will do to your system. You will also be able to determine whether homeopathy is indeed the right

## 9. Homeopathy

treatment for you, or whether you body needs a different form of treatment.

Homeopathy is subtle. It acts like a catalyst, prompting the body to shift how it reacts to an impact or illness. Often it is the body's reaction to an illness rather than the illness itself that causes the most problems. Homeopathy's mechanisms remain a total enigma to us: in truth we have no idea how it works (with our current science knowledge, it should not work) and science has not yet found the right questions to ask, or the right parameters of research to look at it properly. There is also no financial incentive for homeopathy to be looked at properly: homeopathic treatments are cheap to make and therefore millions cannot be made from them. The result of this is that homeopathy is ridiculed, rejected, and ignored by mainstream science.

The major sticking-point with homeopathy, besides its limitations being dependant on the patient's vital force, is that it can be so complex to truly learn how to work with it. I have been studying homeopathy for twenty years and I now realize I have barely scratched the surface. But a basic background knowledge of its key substances, along with an understanding of how the body works with catalysts, vital force and timing, can be invaluable life-saving tools for a magician.

I have used homeopathy very successfully on severely injured or very ill animals, birds, babies, children, magicians, and general folk. I have used it to treat all sorts of complaints, from major head injuries, to magical impacts, to epidemic disease. I have found that a homeopathic treatment can work spectacularly if applied at the right time in the right dose, and work adequately alongside other healing modalities at other times. In the case of magicians with major magical impacts, homeopathy becomes one of the layers of healing applied, rather than the only one. Sometimes, though, a single well-aimed dose can stop something in its tracks: learning how to get to that point of knowledge can take time, however.

The best way for a magician to learn how to use homeopathy magically is to start simply: if you try to give yourself a crash course, nothing will stick; like all deeper dynamics, learning becomes a long path walked at a steady pace, not a two hundred meter dash.

The first steps to take are to obtain a good *Materia Medica*, which is a book of all the substances homeopaths use, their actions, etc. and a *Repertory* (symptoms cross-referenced). I have used a few different *Materia Medica*, and the best I have found by far is *Lotus Materia Medica* by Robin Murphy, ND[1]. It contains a mix of Homeopathy and Spagyric medicines that is detailed, yet clear and concise.

Familiarizing yourself with a few basic remedies, their actions, histories, and applications will give you a starting point. Once you have gained a basic understanding of how these substances operate and have used basic 'first aid' on yourself, then it is time to dip into the *Materia Medica* and look at a chosen substance. There are literally thousands of substances used in homeopathy, but in reality you will only use a few specific ones. I have a stock of about a hundred key remedies in different potencies that I keep and use, and that has sufficed over the years.

As a magician, when you look at different substances, use magical poetic application: if you have been impacted from working with underworld fire magic or have been attacked by such power, then the first step would be to look, via readings, at underworld 'fire' substances like sulphur, phosphorus, or *aurum metallicum* (gold). Gold is heavily linked with dragon power, which in turn is linked with underworld volcanic power. If the magician has been attacked with focused utterance or air magic, then the injury often appears like a 'sword in the back'. That would lead me to look at *hypericum* (St. Johns wort) which is excellent for stab wounds (and head injuries, crushed fingers, etc.). So you begin to see the poetic application of substances in a magical setting.

Now let's look at some key remedies that every magician should have in their home or to hand, and then we will look at how they can be applied, how to take them, and how to work magically with them.

## 9.2 Key remedies

Rather than block this section with too much regular homeopathic information which you can look up in a *Materia Medica*, I will concentrate on the magical uses of substances along with lesser-known 'regular' information and anecdotes. Most of the following remedies have a deep, wide-ranging action upon the

---

[1]R. Murphy (2010). *Lotus Materia Medica*. 3rd ed. Paharganj, New Delhi: B. Jain Publishers (P) Ltd. A repertory by Robin Murphy is also available: R. Murphy (2003). *Homeopathic Medical Repertory: A Clinical and Alphabetical Repertory*. 2nd ed. Blacksburg, Virginia: H. A. N. A. Press.

## 9. Homeopathy

body, and if you are interested in healing, then looking further into these substances with a *Materia Medica* would be very educational.

### 9.3  *Aconitum napellus* (Monkshood)

Essentially, aconite is used when a magician has had the shit scared out of them or sustained a particularly adrenal 'attack.' From a magical perspective, aconite acts directly on the adrenals when they have been pushed into instant overdrive (as opposed to having been worn out). If a dangerous attack is incoming, or the magician has reached too deeply into the inner worlds and has come up against a major destructive being, the body will respond with palpitations, symptoms of panic attack, and a feeling of fear or shock.

Sometimes if an attack comes in at night, the magician can wake up with feelings of foreboding, a fast heart rate, and a sense of being hyper-alert. In these circumstances, taking aconite at a potency of 30c would be helpful.

### 9.4  *Arnica* (Arnica montana)

This is usually the first homeopathic remedy that most people come across. Arnica 'cushions' from minor impact and is most often used for bruising or a 'bruised' feeling. It is a simple remedy, and is used after a heavy vision that has left the magician feeling like they have been moving bricks around for six hours!

For minor magical impact, a bruised feeling, or actual bruises from magical work, Arnica in the 30c potency as a minor acute is usually sufficient to soothe and heal.

### 9.5  *Arsenicum album*

This is a deep–acting, profound remedy that acts on every part of the body. This remedy is a 'must-have' for any magician who does visionary work deep in the inner worlds. The type of incidents that would warrant this remedy are a major physical reaction to angelic work, or the taking-in of knowledge through ingestion.

The major indicators for requiring this remedy are physical: the person is cold and wants to sit almost on top of a fire, or sometimes they feel cold but have a high fever. They may have lower abdominal upsets with burning pains and a burning rectum, dull hair, and/or a pale face with dark rings under their eyes. They may experience complete exhaustion, and be oversensitive and irritable.

When a magician absorbs or encounters a lot of power, it can sometimes send their body into free-fall. If, a few days after the work, their body begins to display symptoms similar to the *arsenicum* description, then this remedy in a 30c would be something to look at.

## 9.6 *Hypericum perforatum* (St. Johns wort)

*Hypericum* in its homeopathic form (and also in its herbal tincture form) is a substance par excellence for magicians and their various injuries. This substance works directly on the brain and nervous system, and it is truly astonishing in its action upon head injuries. Sometimes when too much power is mediated, or a powerful being that is not used to connecting with humans inadvertently causes nervous system damage to someone when they attempt communication, then *hypericum* will restore the fried central nervous system.

Sometimes a homeopathic potency is needed, and other times the herbal tincture itself is best. For immediate 'blast' impacts that are very deep, a higher potency of 1m in a single dose is needed, or repeated doses at 30c (see Choosing Potencies, below). The symptoms that would indicate a need for *hypericum* are either a lasting headache after powerful magical work that does not go away, or a migraine or prolonged, increasing headache that builds over days.

The other condition that this sort of magical impact can trigger is shingles or shingles-type neuralgia in parts of the body, and in such a case *hypericum* (or *rhus tox*) would be indicated. Another thing *hypericum* can be used for magically is to treat magical 'stab' wounds. Sometimes a magician can be attacked using the sword power of utterance, which can appear in the inner body as a stab wound or literally a 'sword in the back'. Taking *hypericum* after magically dealing with such an attack will begin the healing process. This type of attack can appear in the health or directional reading as the Ace of Swords.

Growing St. Johns wort bushes around a house's boundaries will also help to filter such attacks. It will not stop them, but it will lessen the blow.

## 9.7  *Gelsemium*

I call this remedy the 'great awakener,' as that is what it tends to do. Sometimes if a magician reaches too far too deep in vision, they can become 'over-stretched' and lose their anchor in the body. The magician then goes into a slump that goes far beyond fatigue: they cannot open their eyes or they can barely keep them open; they sleep for prolonged periods of time, and are barely conscious.

I did not fully understand the power of this remedy until one day I got to observe its action in a most spectacular way. Even though this is not a magical story, it will demonstrate just how useful this substance can be.

In my thirties I started a rescue for badly injured and traumatized birds. I worked a lot with homeopathy, among other treatments, and the local vet had become deeply impressed with my results. One afternoon, the vet turned up on my doorstep with an unconscious puppy in her arms. She had bought the puppy for her daughter, and on the second round of vaccinations the puppy fell unconscious and slipped into a coma. Three days later, the vet was faced with the prospect of having to euthanize the poor thing, as it looked like the pup was not going to recover.

I did a couple of readings, and pinpointed *gelsemium* in lower (30c) doses. I ground up one dose and placed it inside the pup's gums, and then we waited. Nothing happened. So one hour later, I gave a second dose and told the vet to take the pup home and watch them. They were to give the pup a dose every hour until something happened.

An hour later I had a phone call. A loud yapping could be heard in the background. The pup had woken up during the car ride home and was now racing around the vet's home like a maniac. She was so impressed that she decided to begin the study of homeopathy for her veterinary practice.

*Gelsemium* used at the right time and at the right potency will wake up someone whose energy is trapped or inadvertently shut down. It is not a miracle cure, but it is one of a number of valuable tools that can be used if properly indicated.

## 9.8  Nitric acid

This remedy is very useful to temporarily block the bodily effects of incoming magical attacks. It is not a good idea to use it more than a couple of times in any one period of time, simply because of its magical dynamic: it does not take the magic away; it simply gives your body a bit of respite so that you can tackle the attack yourself. Misused, it will mask the effects of the magic until the attacks have become so powerful that they can overwhelm you.

Use it sparingly when absolutely needed, and ensure that you do readings to look at the longer-term effects. Sometimes we just have to hunker down and deal with an attack, but if you are already sick, weak, or drained, then this remedy can take the pressure off a bit so that you can focus and get to work.

If the body is reacting with the nitric acid symptomatic picture, then it is safe to take it as an acute treatment at 30c every few hours for a day. The picture of physical symptoms to look for is sore or burning cracked corners of the mouth, nose or anus.

## 9.9 Sulphur

The use of sulphur for healing and in magic stretches way back in time, and it can be a brilliant substance to work with magically. Magically, sulphur in its elemental form will attract underworld/demonic forces, and homeopathically it will assist in the job of repelling those same forces from the body. If you have been working deep in the Underworld or the Abyss and come back feeling dirty or sticky, a well-timed dose of sulphur at 30c will help in the clearing process (along with a ritual bath).

If you have become 'sludged' magically and do not realize it, then your body will feel sticky and dirty, you could possibly develop flatulence (yum), red eye rims, and you may break out in spots and generally 'smell.' Sometimes a ritual bath is enough to shift things, but sometimes a dose of sulphur is also needed.

## 9.10 How to take homeopathic remedies (and how to store them)

Homeopathic remedies are best taken when the mouth is clear of tastes and smells. Hence they are taken after thirty minutes of no food or drink, and nothing by mouth for thirty minutes after. Mint (toothpaste or gum) or any strong-smelling substance should not be used at the same time of day as taking the remedy,

## 9. Homeopathy

and avoid anything with strong odours (onions, for example) for two hours before and after taking a remedy.

Perfumes, camphor (tiger balm), and strong-smelling chemicals can cancel out a remedy, and they should not be used on the same day as taking the remedy, and preferably not for a few days after.

Coffee can also cancel many remedies out (it is an antidote), though it has no affect on *arsenicum*. If you are only using a remedy for a day, then stay away from coffee for that day and the subsequent day in order to ensure that the remedy can really get into the body. It is not the caffeine in the coffee; rather it is the coffee itself: decaf will have the same effect as the regular sort.

To take remedies, put the tablet or grains under your tongue and leave them there to melt. If they are hard, crunch them and put the remains under your tongue. Some modern homeopaths will reel off a long list of things you should not eat or drink while working with remedies, but in practice I have not found them to make any difference.

Store your remedies away from heat, light, and strong smells. I have a strong wooden cupboard that all my remedies live in (I have a very large selection), and if properly cared for, they will last for many years.

### 9.11 Choosing the right potency

Choosing the right potency is as important as choosing the right remedy, and taking that remedy at the right time. The basic rule of thumb for general use is as follows: for acute use, or for prolonged treatment over weeks, the lower doses are best. A potency of 30c is perfectly adequate for most purposes, and it is hard for a beginner to do themselves (or anyone else) any damage by using such a potency.

When serious damage has been done, then a higher potency is sometimes needed. The only time not to use a high potency for a serious issue is if the vital force of the person is very low: the higher the potency, the more it pulls on the vital force to initiate a healing crisis and resolution. If the vital force is very low, a high potency can do a lot of damage: under such circumstances, it is better to use other forms of healing such as herbs or acupuncture until the body has a better supply of energy to work with.

For a 'stab' injury from an inner magical attack or a full-on angelic encounter, a dose of *hypericum* at 1m can do a lot of good.

Unless you are experienced in the use of homeopathy, I would not suggest going above 1m in potency. The reason for this is the higher the potency, the deeper into the pattern of the person the remedy goes. A very high potency can change fate patterns and alter how the immune system works, which is often not a good thing to do.

Similarly I have found that potencies below 30c can often aggravate a magical condition without bringing it to resolution. When I was first studying homeopathy, I would do it the traditional way, which is to try and work out the best remedy and potency, and then observe to see what happens. For a very long time it did not occur to me to do health readings first to see whether in fact it was the right remedy and potency.

I did finally discover that it made life a lot easier to actually check if it was the right remedy, potency and dosage; but what also emerged from those readings was a wealth of information as to how the remedies actually worked within the body.

I became able to observe through the readings which potencies would only suppress a condition rather than bring about a 'cure,' which remedies would aggravate things, and which remedies simply moved the symptoms around the body without bringing resolution.

As for timing, in an acute situation take a remedy immediately and then hourly or two hourly for a few doses (check with readings). For a deeper action, it is best to take them at threshold times like dawn or dusk, or at the height of an aggravation. When a deep but subtle shift is needed, particularly if the endocrine system is involved, then taking the remedy as a single dose on a full moon can be very powerful.

For those who are experienced homeopaths, using endocrine sarcodes at the full moon in lower doses (30c) can be very powerful indeed, though caution must be used, as it can drastically alter how a gland operates. If a particular gland has been affected by magic, sometimes it is not the actual gland that needs the remedy; rather it is the 'controller' of that gland that needs the treatment. For example, when the thyroid has been hit by a magical impact, often it is better to treat the pituitary rather than the thyroid.

## 9.12 How remedies work and what to expect

Remedies tend to work from the inside out and from the top down. Take, for example, a magical impact or hit that has

## 9. Homeopathy

affected the internal organs or nervous system and which needs bringing out to the surface. This can be done either through the skin or the emotions. Sometimes a healing crisis will begin to resolve when spots or a rash appears. If that happens, do not suppress the rash: it is better to 'let it all come out'. It is the body's natural clearing mechanism swinging into action, and if you suppress the rash, you also suppress the healing process itself.

Other times the aggravation can express itself through the emotions. If this happens, again do not take anything to suppress the emotional shift: it is better to be bad-tempered, angry, sad, etc. so that the energy dissipates through an emotive crisis. It only becomes a problem if the emotive outlet becomes 'stuck,' and if this happens then further treatment is needed to clear out that emotive expression. Just be aware of what is happening and that the emotion needs to express and release. Warn those close to you, and do not identify with those emotions: just let them flow and wear themselves out.

An interesting dynamic that can also happen with remedies, particularly if the nervous system has taken the magical hit, is that the aggravation will work its way out through the feet or hands. It often happens after the healing crisis has passed: a few days, or even a couple of weeks after taking the remedy, a sharp pain can develop in a foot or toe. Similarly a rash can appear on the foot or hand: this is the CNS clearing out the problem. If this happens, just let it do its job, and it will pass as the body uses its own healing ability to restore balance.

Often the remedies used to clear a magical impact bring on a minor 'crisis' or initial aggravation of symptoms before resolution. This is normal, and unless it continues, it should be left alone. Other times, particularly if the person's vital force is healthy, a well-timed remedy can simply and quietly resolve an impact. When the healing is almost complete, often a spot or boil will appear, or a small rash, or they will have a day of crying: it is as though the body gathers up the magical impact and pushes it out of the body. It is truly fascinating to see this in action.

Another even more fascinating dynamic to see in action is a very strange but powerful display of time/energy shifts that can be triggered by remedies. When the magician is struggling hard under the weight of an attack or impact, and the correct remedy and dosage is chosen, a remarkable thing can happen: upon the moment of choosing the right action, the symptoms vanish—even before the remedy is taken. But if the magician then decides they are not going to take the remedy after all, the symptoms come back.

I have come across skilled homeopaths that would treat a patient by choosing the right substance and dosage, and then just have the patient hold the remedy rather than actually take it. I have never been able to achieve that myself, but I have seen it in action and it is truly astonishing. It is not a psychosomatic healing as I have seen this also done with animals, by simply choosing the right remedy and then projecting that choice towards the suffering or injured animal. It is a truly magical skill, and is very rare, but it is impressive to watch when it is done by someone adept at working at that level. The healing seems to happen in the inner landscape of the person, which in turn triggers the body into action.

## 9.13 Demons/disease consciousness and nosodes

Something I stumbled upon quite by accident was that certain disease nosodes can help to clear or protect against the beings that flow through those diseases. A nosode is a homeopathic preparation made from diseased tissue, pus, blood, and other discharges. I had already come across what I call 'hive' consciousnesses within some diseases, and they would be labelled as 'demonic forces' by some.

When I was doing a lot of work in the inner desert (the Tree of Life is a map of this desert) I noticed that some forces, which were destructive forms of consciousness, would embed themselves in certain large patterns that would then flow out into the world. I spent some time observing, following, and attempting to interact with these forces to learn more about them.

Over time I came to observe these forces as they crossed into Malkuth and watched as they expressed themselves as epidemics in animals and humans. They seemed to have a variety of functions, and some of those functions were very surprising.

Not only did they cull or weaken, but they also seemed to change the consciousness of the human or animal that they infected. I was fascinated. The implications for this could be huge: if a virus or bacterial infection can radically change how a population expresses itself intellectually and emotionally, that in turn would change that society's culture.

## 9. Homeopathy

This was the beginning for me of a much wider understanding of how demonic forces work out in the world, and what their various functions were in the larger scheme of things. I was already aware of how the use of metals and precious stones, mined and brought to the surface, could shift how a society functioned - lead, gold, tin, copper for example can have a profound effect upon the brain through constant exposure: we now know that chronic lead exposure can cause aggression. But it had not occurred to me that infections within populations could also shift how that population functioned. From a medical perspective it is fascinating, and is something that is only just being looked at by science. If a virus infects a large portion of the population and is not deadly (herpes for example), but shifts how the brain, nervous system, immune system and endocrine system works, then you have a changed society.

From a magical perspective, we see this as various forces flowing in and out of the world in an attempt to restore equilibrium in the balance of creation and destruction. This also leads onto a discussion of inherited disease patterns. Certain infectious diseases cause a permanent shift in how the immune system works. That shift is then inherited by subsequent generations, which in turn slowly brings about a change in how the human body reacts to disease in general. This can potentially bring about changes to a society, particularly if that immune change affects the mind and emotions. Certain diseases can literally 'change the world' for humans.

This can be a good or bad thing, but it is probably a bit of both. Like the outer manifestation of certain diseases, the inner pattern or consciousness of a disease can 'prime' our inner immune systems against much larger and more dangerous intrusions, so they should not be necessarily considered to be a danger.

Back to the magical importance of this topic. If the magician is working down the Abyss or deep in the Underworld, then there is a chance that at some point they will bump up against one of the beings that manifests through disease. If they are deep down the Abyss, then the chances are that the disease they manifest through is extinct or almost removed from humanity. Anything down the Abyss is in a process of moving away from the manifest world. The further down the Abyss a being is, the longer they have been out of circulation.

When you come across these beings, it is often because you are being asked to help 'seal them up' or bind them further down the Abyss. In the process of such work, the magician can become 'infected' by the being and as a result become ill. This is where homeopathic nosodes come into their own. Once an inner infection has been triggered by these beings, particularly if their disease expression is a virus, you can never really get rid of it, but you can keep it dormant through the use of nosodes.

If after such work you find yourself coming down with an illness, look to the symptomatic picture that presents itself. If it is a simple illness from overstretching yourself or a basic impact, then treat it accordingly. If, however, you start to get strange symptoms, then it is not that you have caught the disease itself from the being; it is more a matter of your body manifesting the disease pattern. The body reacts to the inner being as it had been fully infected.

One such incident that happened to me had my doctor fascinated. After some deep work down the Abyss I developed a fever, horrific back pain, and a large single pustule deeply embedded in my skin (like a smallpox pustule—chickenpox, which I have already had, sits on top of the skin; smallpox embeds itself into the skin). The pustule was photographed by the doctor, samples taken, blood tests, etc., which all came back negative, and my doctor was stumped. I took a smallpox nosode (*variolinum*) and the symptoms settled within hours. The pustule left a little scar, and I was left with a lot to think about.

In such cases, treatment with the disease nosode at a potency of 30c will nudge the body to normality, and will cancel out the body's reaction. If you intend to work deeply in the Abyss, then it would be wise to familiarize yourself with the symptomatic picture of some of the deadlier diseases, and have a small bottle of each one's nosodes to hand.

## 9.14 Summary

In terms of medicine that works energetically, homeopathy is second to none. If your hit was a deep energetic one and the body struggles under the weight of such power, then homeopathy should be the first thing you look at in terms of a treatment reading. When you do a health reading to choose a homeopathic remedy, do not simply look at the short-term effect; look at the long-term effect too.

Some remedies can bring about healing in the short-term but wreak havoc in the longer-term: many powerful remedies can keep working for a long time, so bear that in mind.

## 9. Homeopathy

When you do a health reading to choose a remedy, it is important to see if the vital components of the body would be brought back into balance. So you are looking for balanced or regenerative cards in the inner landscape, the head, the vital organs, the sexual organs, and the longer-term immune system. If aggravating cards appear in the position of the lower intestines or skin, but everything else is fine, then it shows you the route that the body will use to process the problem: expect a tummy upset, runny butt, or a rash as the body clears itself out.

If you wish to experiment and learn through using readings, a good way to do that would be to choose a group of remedies and look at the effects that each one would have on your body. It will teach you a lot about how the substances work, and how your unique body works to process issues. You will see how, with the right remedy, the body pushes the aggravation away from the vital organs and brain in a centrifugal pattern, whereas an illness brought about by one of those deep Abyssal beings tends to affect the body in a centripetal pattern; it attacks from the outside in, with the symptoms inching their way to your centre.

Always look for a centrifugal pattern in the reading, with the problems on the periphery and the healing in the centre and the head. Also look closely at the relationship between the small intestine and the brain: make sure that if the lower intestine is aggravated, it is not affecting the brain. If it is, then you need to find a remedy that will use a different route.

A lot of this information can be overwhelming for someone who is new to Homeopathy, but don't try to bog yourself down with too much irrelevant information: simply learn the very basic remedies for emergency use, and take it from there. As you progress and explore more, you can revisit this text and learn a little bit more: take everything a step at a time.

Chapter Ten

# *Herbs and Substances*

## 10.1 Just a spoonful of sugar

Herbs are another great tool to have handy in your emergency 'I have just blown myself up' kit. Like Homeopathy, there are thousands of various herbal remedies to choose from, but in practice you will find that a small group of herbs work just fine for you and your needs. What can work well for some will not work well for others, and so like every other form of treatment, it is about learning what your body needs—and does not need—to aid healing.

Before you take anything, do a reading to see whether the herb will be useful to you or not, and remember that what worked for a past disaster will not necessarily be the best thing for the current meltdown. Learning to be flexible with how you approach your own healing is vital. Also check to see if a herb is compatible with any medication you are currently taking, and let your doctor know you are taking herbs. Some can interfere with your medication.

Herbs are generally used to treat magical illness or injury when the vital force of the person is in reasonable (or even poor) condition, and the impact or injury did not go too far in. They are also very useful when the body does not need a deep shift, but something more on the surface yet strong-acting, something that will work directly on the organs themselves. Homeopathy reaches into the inner patterns strongly while affecting the outer body; herbs reach the organs and tissues directly and strongly while only nudging the inner energy.

Sometimes herbs and homeopathy can follow each other nicely, and it is always wise to consider a shift from one to the other if necessary. Herbs are also excellent for long-term repair. Once the homeopathy has gone in and started the repair process at a deep level, the herbs can then start the mop-up process, restoring the body's strength and giving it the tools it needs to begin proper repair and rebalancing.

## 10. Herbs and Substances

Herbs can also act as long-term support for the system when the body is going through massive changes like menopause, or through prolonged stress like divorce or bereavement. Herbs are also a good support if you are undertaking long-term, difficult magical service: they uphold the integrity of your system while it is under stress and stops your body buckling under pressure.

Let's look at the action of various herbs on specific areas of the body, as that is probably the easiest approach. As there are literally thousands of potential herbs that can be used, I am not going to block this chapter up with pages and pages of them; rather I will outline a select few that I have used successfully in various magical situations. From there you can do more research for yourself, find out what grows near where you live, and also learn how to grow and work with your own herbs.

Some of the ones I have listed may not be right for you, but they will give you a starting point to work from. As with all herbs, little and often is the best approach, particularly with long-term treatment. Do not get into the silly mentality of 'more is better'—you can overwhelm or even poison your body by taking too much of anything.

Think subtle, and build from there. There will also come a point, particularly with taking a herb over weeks or months, where continuing begins to become counterproductive: when the body has had enough, it will tell you. Be sensitive to your body's reactions, and be willing to flow with the tides of healing. The following groups are the most common areas in the body for magical injury and impact.

### 10.2 Head and brain

When too much power is mediated, or communion happens with a being that is very powerful or not used to communicating with humans, often a head injury can manifest. This can range from intense headaches, migraines, or dizziness, up to a full manifestation of concussion. Tinnitus or earache is also common after a powerful interaction—the nerve branch that feeds the ear, eye and teeth on one side of the face can become impacted from a powerful communication, causing the nerve to become inflamed.

The first line of herbal treatment for any head impact is St. Johns wort. This substance is truly the magician's best friend, as it works directly on the brain and central nervous system. However it is a powerful herb, and if you are on any type of medication

## 10.2. Head and brain

it is wise to check that St. Johns wort does not interact with it. Most importantly of all, if you are on any form of antidepressant, you must not take St. Johns wort at all: you could end up with serotonin syndrome, a deadly condition, as this herb raises your serotonin levels.

St. Johns wort is best taken in tincture form (tincture in grain alcohol is best, as it has a long shelf life), by putting the drops under your tongue. If you suffer from intense or increasing headaches after powerful magical work, take a few drops of this tincture morning and night until it passes. If the headache is intense, then try a few drops every hour until it starts to fade, and continue to take the tincture morning and night for two or three days.

The other substance par excellence for intense headaches, particularly migraines, is feverfew. If you find yourself the victim of a massive migraine after magical work, then taking feverfew in tincture form, using the same method as for St. Johns wort, will usually get rid of it. As with all things to do with magic and the body, you should decide the best approach by looking through a health reading to see which herb the body will respond to best without causing any side-effects.

Feverfew is not for everyone, and should be treated with respect: it is a powerful substance, and too much of it will cause a headache. It is also a blood thinner, so that needs taking into account when making choices. If you are already on blood thinners, taking feverfew would be a bad idea.

Both St. Johns wort and feverfew taste like shit in tincture form, but that is the best way to take them. If you find you don't want to take them because of the taste, then you need to grow some balls. If a little bit of 'uncomfortable' scares you off, then you should not be doing deep magic!

Another good substance to take is cod liver oil. This is not an emergency substance, but rather a healthy maintenance substance that will protect your brain and central nervous system from long-term energetic bumps and knocks. We spend a lot of time indoors and get very little direct sunlight, particularly those of us who live in the more northern countries.

Vitamin D, which the body makes from exposure to sunlight and/or fish oils, is central to a healthy brain and nervous system. A daily dose of cod liver oil, particularly in fall, winter and spring, when sunlight is not so good and people tend to spend more time indoors, will help to keep you strong and on your

## 10. Herbs and Substances

feet. Different forms of delivery are available, and capsules are probably the kindest way to take it.

*Avena sativa* (oatstraw) tincture is a good tonic for the central nervous system, and can really help to put a magician back on their feet if they have taken a bit of a hammering. It soothes and nourishes the nervous system, as well as helps to build back strength. If after a major round of magic you feel frazzled, drained, and generally headache-prone, but not fatigued enough to use St. Johns wort, then consider using Avena tincture (or eat a bowl of oats every day).

### 10.3  Heart impact

If a magician undertakes a long and dangerous magical service task, especially if they are older, then it is possible that they may take a heart impact. Usually such an impact is more inner than outer, but left unattended it can eventually express itself through the physical heart.

In such cases, the first port of call is working directly with the heart and heart guardian in vision. The follow up to this visionary healing can consist of the use of two different herbs: motherwort, or hawthorn. Personally I have always found motherwort to be better and my body responds very well to it. But I have found that for some other magicians, hawthorn was better. Again, it is back to doing a reading to see what treatment would work best.

Motherwort is a powerful and very magical herb in all respects. It strengthens both the heart and the general constitution, and it is deeply connected to the lion goddesses like Sekhmet. I have found that it is best to take it in tincture form, particularly if you also work magically with Sekhmet to 'charge' the tincture. It is also good for priestesses when they approach or are in the midst of menopause and when they are under a great deal of strain. Taking a few drops in the morning and in the evening for a while is a good idea when the magician needs restoration and strengthening.

Hawthorn is best taken the same way, in tincture form, and a simple reading should outline to the magician which herb is better to use.

## 10.4 Bone, joint and muscle injuries

Sometimes when you grapple with inner beings you can acquire physical injuries. Minor dislocations, bruising, hairline fractures, and soft tissue injuries are not uncommon when dealing with larger beings deep in the inner worlds (think Jacob wrestling with angels). When such struggles are described in the Bible, the story is often assumed to be allegorical. It is not, as any magician who has worked closely with inner beings will tell you: such injuries are very real and very possible.

These injuries do not mean that you have been 'fighting' with angelic beings; rather it is the sheer power they pack during communication that often brings about injury. I have had a few very painful injuries from grappling/conversing with beings. If such injuries are not attended to properly, they can leave a permanent weakness in a joint.

If you do acquire such an injury in vision, ensure that you work on it using visionary healing as well as direct application of herbal compounds: both the inner and the outer injury will need fixing.

The first line of treatment for such injuries is a comfrey compress. This plant is extraordinary in its healing abilities, and it grows easily in temperate climates. It does have some warnings attached, however, as this is a powerful plant.

Never take comfrey internally, and do not use it on broken skin: it can affect your liver if you have liver disease, and it is readily absorbed through the skin. So do not use comfrey if you have liver disease! It is best used on injuries like fractures, sprains, pulled or impacted muscles, ligament tears, sprains, etc.

If it is to be used on ligament tears or fractures, make sure that the position of the limb has been set before applying the comfrey: the herb speeds up the setting process considerably, so you want to make sure that everything is where it is supposed to be! It is perfect for use with these types of injuries if you have a removable splint: you can take the split off, apply the poultice, and then re-splint.

To make a comfrey compress/poultice, see the section in this chapter headed 'poultice'. During the first two days of the injury, once the poultice has cooled down put it back in the pan to reheat it and repeat the application. This should be done four or five times a day for the first couple of days, and then twice a day thereafter for four or more days.

## 10. Herbs and Substances

For less drastic injuries, such as aching or minor pulled muscles, arnica cream, comfrey cream, or *Ruta graveolens* cream would suffice. *Ruta graveolens* (common rue) is a very interesting herb, and one that can also be used in homeopathic form. It has a direct action on ligaments and tendons, and it is particularly good for tendonitis or small joint strain. In herbal form it is best used as a cream (but not internally), but it can also be taken homeopathically for pain and injury.

As an aside, common rue is an excellent herb to grow along your property's boundary or to hang over the inside of your door: it has interesting qualities that certain beings do not like, and it is well known in folk magic as a threshold protector.

### 10.5 Skin neuralgia

Sometimes inner impacts or injuries can manifest as a burning or stinging pain on the skin. Sometimes this can be so bad that it is like having a poison ivy rash without the rash, or like having shingles. Essentially, the nerve endings have been 'injured' or aggravated by an inner impact, and one of the best treatments I have found for that is *Rhus toxicodendron* cream.

It is a preparation made from a dilution of poison ivy, and it is one of the substances that bridges between herbal and homeopathic use. It is good to have in your first aid kit, but it is best not to overuse it, as it can irritate the skin if it is used when it is not necessary.

### 10.6 Burns

Burns or burning sensations are another common side-effect of working with too much power, or of going deep into the Underworld or too far out in the stars. It is not uncommon to come out of vision and find you have 'sunburn' on your face or arms.

I always keep a bottle of Aloe vera in the fridge, or some of its large leaves in the freezer for such occasions, now that I grow the plant. Smearing the Aloe juice on the red areas takes them down very quickly. It is second to none as a treatment for any form of burn, be it magical or otherwise. The close second would be calendula tincture dabbed on the red skin. If the skin is broken, then add the tincture to cooled boiled water and wash the wound regularly and carefully.

## 10.7 Endocrine imbalances and the menopause

The endocrine system operates a very delicate balancing act that can be knocked out of whack by magical work. Herbs are one of the ways that a magician can restore balance within the body, or at least support the endocrine system as it rebalances itself.

We notice when our system is out of balance because we become tired, drained, emotional, or feel brain-fogged. When such symptoms continue for any length of time, it is possible that magic has affected some part of this delicate and complex system within our bodies.

As we get into our late forties and onwards, the body goes through a number of changes, the most spectacular of which for both men and women are the menopause and perimenopausal transition. Menopause is a natural process, and it affects individuals in many different ways and to different degrees. When you throw powerful magic into the mix, the effects can become more pronounced.

Not only does our hormone system go into free-fall, but the menopause can also affect our ability to deal with stress, and for a magician this can become a major problem.

Magic of any real power causes physical and emotional stress, and the massive changes that magic can produce in our daily lives also brings a great deal of stress into our minds and bodies. If this is not properly dealt with it can cause a major upheaval in our endocrine system, and it is important to be attentive to such effects and treat them accordingly. Some magicians sail through this period of change with little ill effect, whereas others are not so lucky.

The menopause is also a time when working practice should be adjusted to take account of such hormone shifts. It also tends to coincide with an interesting dynamic that many magicians have reported to me, and that I have experienced for myself. It is that the older and more experienced a magician you become, the more power you can output through simple magical action.

An adept will find that their regular magical practice fades when they reach their late forties and fifties, and a different power dynamic kicks in: you do less magic overall, but when you do act magically, a huge amount of power comes through. This is the time of your life when you really learn that less is more, and that inner magical action should only be used when absolutely necessary.

## 10. Herbs and Substances

It is also a time when, for magicians well versed in visionary magic, outer magical actions automatically trigger deep inner shifts: after decades of visionary work, the magician evolves from working deep in vision to simple outer triggers that engage deep inner resources. A simple ritual action that would have had no effect whatsoever in your twenties can trigger a massive power shifts in your later years: as the inner pathway is already established, all that is needed is the outer catalyst.

Along with this transition often come issues with the endocrine system, as we learn to slowly disengage from inner power actions and instead engage outer power actions. Those endocrine issues can manifest in a variety of ways, as our bodies struggle to deal with the outer change and inner shift. How they affect any one magician will largely depend on what they are working with, what inner energy resources have already been depleted, and how their bodies are adapting to the shift.

Over the last decade, I have come across a variety of herbs that have helped enormously with these tidal changes, but a word of caution before I discuss them: most of these herbs are powerful and should be treated with respect. Do not take them indiscriminately: look closely through readings and body observations to ensure that you choose the appropriate herb, and only take it when necessary. Properly chosen and sensibly taken, these herbs can help you through this transition and ensure that you emerge out the other end in one piece. Often the body can rebalance itself if it is given time; if you dive in suddenly with tons of herbs it is likely that you will create more chaos as opposed to triggering healing.

Endocrine-active herbs can also be very useful for younger magicians in their thirties who have drained their inner resources or who have suffered illness or major stresses that have left them with fatigue, depression, or just plain run them down.

Sometimes powerful work clashes with the surges of hormones that magicians encounter in their twenties and thirties, and this clash of hormonal power versus magical power can create an upheaval in the mind and body which can be very difficult to deal with.

The first action for rebalancing from such an upheaval is emotional and physical self-discipline: these power surges can come in the form of heightened sex drives, or strong emotional swings, intense cravings, etc. Your reaction to your first dose of real magical power will determine how you develop as a magician in the future.

Instead of succumbing to 'emotive drama' or a rampant sex drive, the first step is to recognize what is happening. That step alone can take time to sink in. It is one thing to recognize it intellectually; it is quite another to really understand it and be able to act upon it.

Often that first stage is successfully navigated one step at a time. For me it was a very difficult time as I was full of both aggressive hormones and magical power. Step by step I managed to slow down and view what was happening. From there, it was a slow walk of self-discipline, homeopathy, herbs, and a shift in my magical practice which enabled me to tiptoe my way through it. It was not pleasant and I frazzled a few folks along the way, but eventually I learned how to balance my power and body together.

Once emotive self-discipline is established, you will begin to see how your pattern of emotional behaviour relates to magical acts and bodily reactions. Once you can see what's going on, herbs and homeopathy can be used to help with the process. Recognizing the magical triggers and traps that are endemic to the magical path is important: your twenties and thirties is the time of your life when the messiah trap opens in front of you. See it, recognize it, and side-step it.

The following herbs can be used to address minor endocrine imbalances brought about by magical work. If the symptoms are severe, then seeing a doctor is the recommended route: when the endocrine system is seriously out of balance then trying to treat it yourself is folly. Such severe imbalance can kill you or leave permanent damage: when in doubt, go to your doctor!

## 10.8 St. Johns wort (*Hypericum perforatum*)

The magician's friend and a substance you should be familiar with by now (it has been mentioned enough in this book!). Magical work can really knock the serotonin levels in your body, leaving you feeling fatigued, fogged, and depressed. The tincture of the herb taken twice daily should make a massive difference. It is also one of the few substances that can be used as a prophylactic: take it before the heavy magical work so that it acts as a buffer against impact.

This substance can also come in useful when the magician is in the midst of the youthful power/drama/imbalance phase.

## 10. Herbs and Substances

Carefully used (if indicated in readings), this tincture can slowly 'ground' the magician enough for them to be able to use their own focus and mental discipline to bring things under control.

### 10.9 Siberian Ginseng (*Eleutherococcus senticosus*)

This is another adaptogen that can help the body cope with magical impact. It is also what I call the great indicator: I have found that when it is taken, it will often bring any underlying physical problems to the surface, so that they can be spotted and treated.

If the fatigue of the magician is due to a slow-burn infection, then E. senticosus will bring that infection right out by triggering an immune response. If the fatigue is caused by a magical impact to the serotonin and/or dopamine levels, E. senticosus will often nudge things back to normal within a week of taking it.

It is best used as a preventative, taken before heavy magical work and then again directly after the work is finished. It is not something that should be taken as a long-term supplement, simply because the body can adapt to it and it will stop working within a few weeks. If the magician's inner energy stores are depleted, then taking E. senticosus for more than a few days will begin to drain whatever is left of those precious resources.

### 10.10 Kelp (*Laminaria*)

Kelp is a good source of iodine, a chemical element which is necessary for many vital functions in the body, including keeping the thyroid healthy. In some countries like the USA, iodine is added to table salt, so these populations do not really need to take kelp supplements. The rest of us can become deficient in iodine from time to time, and if magical work is affecting the thyroid gland (common in women magicians), then it may be appropriate to take kelp.

As with any powerful substance, do a health reading first to see if your body really needs it, as taking kelp unnecessarily can cause thyroid issues. Kelp should not be taken if you have a tendency for an overactive thyroid (it will speed it up more) and if you are not sure, speak to your doctor. Also be aware that often Kelp can have widely fluctuating levels of iodine in it. Sometimes simply taking vitamins that have a daily recommended dose of iodine included is sufficient.

## 10.11 Velvet bean (*Mucuna pruriens*)

This is an interesting Ayurvedic herb that has a direct action on a body's dopamine levels. Sometimes certain forms of magic can knock out the sensitive balance of various neurotransmitters in the body, and dopamine is one that is easily knocked out.

The symptomatic picture that would warrant the use of this herb is fatigue, problems staying in a deep sleep, low sex drive, poor muscle action, tremors, and the physical effects of stress. It works strongly on the central nervous system, and is a tonic for nerves, muscles, and the reproductive system.

It is not wise to take it long-term, but it would probably be helpful for a month or so if the magician has taken a heavy knock. It can raise the blood pressure, and it is not a good herb for someone to take who has manic, depressive or psychotic tendencies (but people suffering such illnesses should also not be doing magic). As with any powerful herb, look it up, check it does not clash with any medication you are taking, and do a health reading to see if it would help you.

## 10.12 Shatavari (*Asparagus racemosus*)

Another Ayurvedic herb, Shatavari is of particular help to women magicians who are starting to notice menopausal symptoms, and young female magicians who are suffering from burnout. Like all herbs, it is not a wonder-drug or cure-all, but it can make a real difference by helping to smooth down the various hormonal upsets that happen as women approach and then are immersed in menopause. It is also excellent for overworked young women who are drained physically, magically, and emotionally.

## 10.13 Ashwagandha (*Withania somnifera*)

This is a good herb from India that really helps the brain, nervous system and endocrine system get back on track after a magical impact. It is a calm, regenerative herb that strengthens while soothing a system that has been knocked out of balance by magical action or attack. It is not gentle, however, and like

## 10. Herbs and Substances

most Ayurvedic herbs it needs to be treated with some respect. It seems to work better for men than women, though that is not a hard and fast rule.

### 10.14 Chamomile (*Matricaria chamomilla, Chamaemelum nobile*)

Chamomile is an often-overlooked herb as it is so easily available: people think it is gentle and therefore of no real use. It is a mistake to underestimate chamomile's action. It was well-known to the ancient Egyptians, and used in a wide rage of applications by their temple priests.

This herb is wonderful for navigating through the disruptive power, emotional and magical upheavals that we hit in our late twenties and early thirties. It is a calming herb, is anti inflammatory, and brings with it a subtle strengthening power to frazzled minds and bodies.

Taking it as a tincture, or drinking it regularly and daily as a steeped tea can be very useful when our hormone systems go crazy. It can be used for many months and will slowly calm things down, which in turn enables the magician to engage their own self-healing.

### 10.15 Anti-inflammatory herbs

Another side-effect of magic that can sometimes hit a magician is inflammation. This often happens when you are dealing with powerful beings and the body's immune system reacts to your inner interactions as though the body is physically being invaded: it triggers an inflammatory reaction that can then spread throughout the body.

Sometimes specific 'weak' areas of the body will respond with inflammation, and I have found that herbs can help to calm things down. It can be anything from an inflamed joint, to gastrointestinal inflammation, to more generalized inflammatory reactions.

A good substance I found that helped was turmeric. I use turmeric in cooking quite a lot, and it can also be taken in capsule form when needed. The whole dynamic of inflammation in the body is complex and not fully understood from a medical perspective, so do not think that it can be treated easily or lightly.

Something which I observed repeatedly with magicians who suffered from bouts of inflammation as a result of magical work was that ordinary inflammatory drugs seemed to 'back up' the inflammation expression in the body. The drug would lessen the inflammation briefly, but as soon as it was stopped, the inflammation would return in double strength.

After having similar experiences myself, I turned to using diet and turmeric as a gentler but effective approach. This will not work for everyone, but it is something to consider and experiment with.

The other anti-inflammatory herb I came upon is Boswellia (frankincense). This is an interesting mix of a magical substance and a healing herb. When I have an inflammatory reaction to magical work, Boswellia often helps calm things down. I use it in capsule form, and I also chew good-quality Frankincense resin.

## 10.16 Protective herbs for the land

Another interesting way for a magician to work with herbs is to grow them and spend time around them. Many herbs have protective qualities in terms of magical boundaries upon the land, and although they will not stop a magical attack, they will filter off some of its power as it comes towards you.

Many of these herbs subtly change the energy of the land around you, and part of a magician's work is to tend to and connect with the land around their home. Some of these herbs discourage inner 'pests,' and if you are sensitive enough you can also work with them in communion: building a relationship with certain plants can act as an early warning mechanism. The group consciousness of the plant's species becomes tuned into you and visa versa, so that when trouble comes barrelling over the horizon it will 'tweak' your radar.

Each country has its own historical tradition of working with plants, not just to take into oneself, but also to protect an area or household. This is a symbiotic relationship whereby the human feeds the plant and tends it, and the plant interacts with the human. Some of the plants I have around my garden are poisonous and very magical, and others are medicinal and also magical.

Growing and harvesting your own medicinal plants is also a very interesting process, as it enables you to slowly learn how to discern the best times for harvesting, the times to nurture, and the times to leave the plant in peace. Making sure the plants

## 10. Herbs and Substances

are fed with good quality organic fertilizer is very important, and also letting other 'weeds' grow around them. Weeds that are not allowed to run riot can 'buddy up' to weaker, more delicate plants, and offer strength and protection to them.

If you have a garden or a patch of land, watch carefully to see how the magical plant affects the other plants around it; that will teach you a lot about its magical and medicinal qualities.

### 10.17   Useful garden herbs for magic or medicine

| | |
|---|---|
| *St. John's wort* | *Hypericum perforatum* |
| *Comfrey* | *Symphytum officinale* |
| *Self-heal* | *Prunella vulgaris* |
| *Henbane* | *Hyoscamus niger* |
| *Wild teasel* | *Dipsacus fullonum* |
| *Holly* | *Ilex aquifolium* |
| *Common hawthorn* | *Crataegus monogna* |
| *Rue* | *Ruta graveolens* |
| *Stinging nettle* | *Urtica dioica* |
| *Common wormwood, mugwort* | *Artemisia vulgaris* |
| *Grand wormwood* | *Artemisia absinthium* |
| *Foxglove* | *Digitalis purpurea* |
| *Tansy* | *Tanacetum vulgare* |
| *Lobelia, Indian tobacco* | *Lobelia inflata* |
| *Marigold* | *Calendula officinalis* |
| *Common broom* | *Cytisus scoparius* |
| *Bramble, blackberry bush* | *Rubus fruticosus* |
| *Motherwort, lion's tail* | *Leonurus cardiaca* |

These herbs and plants all grow in English gardens. If you live in a very different climate, it is worth doing some research to find out what local plants operate in a similar way so that you can work as much as possible with natives or established incomers.

The good boundary-keepers of the above list are St. Johns wort, motherwort, henbane, holly, bramble, rue and hawthorn. Hanging a bunch of rue over the inside of the front door is a very old protective folk tradition. Rue is a powerful herb and is an irritant: always use gloves when handling it.

Henbane is a great plant to sleep around during summer: it is a plant you make friends with, but also treat with a great deal of respect. Henbane is poisonous and should not be taken

## 10.17. Useful garden herbs for magic or medicine

internally, but hanging out with it and sleeping alongside it has some interesting magical effects.

The sleeping technique can be used with a lot of poisonous plants that affect the mind: in California I used to sleep around *Datura stramonium* and *Brugmansia* bushes get to know the plants in my dreams. This technique builds up a very subtle relationship with the plant, and sidesteps the need to risk poisoning yourself by ingestion.

Foxgloves are good strong early warning systems, as is a bush of broom and a patch of *lobelia*. *Lobelia* is a good plant to sit next to while working with magical utterance: it seems to help strengthen and focus your use of breath.

From the plants listed above, good medicinal ones to learn how to work with are St. Johns wort, motherwort, hawthorn, tansy, teasel, marigold, self-heal, comfrey and stinging nettle. Medicinally, some of the herbs are harvested for their roots, others for their flowers and leaves, and in some cases the whole plant can be used: self-heal, for instance. Self-heal is a good wound-wash, an anti–inflammatory, and can be used as a herbal drink, an ointment, or a compress. It is excellent for wounds and minor injuries.

Stinging nettle is a wonderful herb. They are great boundary–keepers, they enrich the land, and they help to strengthen a person after a long winter. Spring nettle leaves can be used for tea, or to put in cooking and to hang around the house for protection. Use gloves for harvesting, and take only the small young leaves (the older larger ones are bitter). They can be put fresh into a stew like spinach, or washed and put into a pot of boiling water for tea. Nettles are full of vitality, vitamins, and inner energy.

Teasel and comfrey are mainly harvested for their roots. We have already discussed comfrey earlier in the chapter, so let's have a look at wild teasel. This plant is astonishing in its vitality and vigour. Its root is an excellent antiviral, and has a very good reputation for treating Lyme's Disease. It is also a helpful magical plant used in tincture form for someone who has been 'invaded' by parasites or other low-level inner beings. Teasel tincture (yuck) helps to strengthen a body that has been weakened by inner attack or invasion, and will help to repair the body's own boundary system.

Teasel must be harvested before it shoots up its main stem, so look for the ground plant which usually grows wild all over the place. I let the flower stems grow, as the whole flowering

## 10. Herbs and Substances

plant is a great land protector. I harvest only a small number of the plants for their roots, and let the rest grow wild around my garden.

Motherwort and hawthorn are both great heart strengtheners, as well as being protective of the land. Their leaves and flowers can be used as teas or made into tinctures, and both of these herbs have powerful actions on the health of the heart.

Dried marigold flowers (*calendula*) are wonderfully soothing when used topically on the skin (great for burns) and to treat inflammation. I use the tincture for sore gums, burns and inflamed skin, and calendula cream is awesome for the skin in general.

### 10.18 Using your own herbs

If you grow your own herbs either in the garden or in pots, or forage for them out in the countryside, what then? What you do with them depends upon what you need them for.

Do not forget to tell the plant that you intend to take some of it, which gives it the chance to be ready and not be taken unawares. Strange as it sounds, this does make a difference. It is also something that happens in nature between trees and plants: if an infestation, fire, or a lot of harvesting is underway, the trees and plants signal each other in a chain of communication that can spread for miles. Also remember to take only what you need, and take bits from different plants, not all the leaves from one plant.

Some herbs are best harvested at the full moon; some are better at the new moon. Some need harvesting just before they go into main bloom. Each herb acts in a different way in terms of their potency. Look up the harvesting details for each plant before you decide to harvest them.

### 10.19 House protection: making bundles

If you are gathering herbs to protect your home and hang around the house in bunches, then collect them just before the peak of the full moon in late spring or early summer, when they will be at their strongest. Remember to use gloves, as most of the protective herbs can also be poisonous, or at least irritant.

For protective use, simply bundle the herbs together with string and hang over doors, beds and windows. You will need to renew them every couple of months and place the old ones in the fire or on the compost heap. The best bundles are rue, motherwort, St. Johns wort and sage.

Henbane wrapped with broom is good for over the bed, as is rue mixed with mugwort. Mugwort is safe to use as a smudging plant, and can be mixed with sage to burn around the house. Rue is *not* safe to burn—its presence in the house is enough.

## 10.20  Infusions

If you need a medicinal herb of reasonable strength and it is the leaves or flowers that are medicinal, then using the infusion method is very good. To make an infusion, gather enough fresh leaves to three-quarters fill a saucepan, and pour in enough filtered water to cover the leaves. Put on a lid, bring the mix to the boil, and let it boil for a couple of minutes. Then turn the heat down to low, and let the mix simmer for a couple of minutes before turning off the heat. Leave the lid on, and let the mix sit and steep for ten to twelve hours.

At the end of steeping, strain the fluid into a jar. This is your infusion. It should be kept in the fridge and used a cup at a time, once in the morning and once in the evening. For more powerful herbs, use a small four-ounce cup twice a day, and for weaker or more nourishing herbs like nettle, drink a few cups a day as and when you need it. This method can also be used with dried herbs, and if you need a strong infusion, then dried herbs are best.

## 10.21  Tinctures

Making your own tinctures from plants is easy and can save you a lot of money. I have found that brandy is the best alcohol to use for tinctures, but many people use gin, whisky or vodka: whatever you use, it needs to be at least 40% proof.

Working with dried herbs is best for making tinctures, and all you need is a bag of the dried herbs, a bottle of 40% proof alcohol, and a good-sized jar with a strong seal that has been cleaned and sterilized.

When I make them, if I am using fresh herbs, I fill the jar with the fresh herbs but don't push them down. When using dried herbs, I half fill the jar with the dried herbs, and fill up the jar with alcohol. Seal the jar well and give it a good shake. Put it on a shelf where you can easily access it, and every day when you walk past, pick it up and give it a good shake. Keep it out of

## 10. Herbs and Substances

direct sunlight, and make sure you label it (you will forget what it is, particularly if you are doing more than one herb at a time).

Let the mixture sit for two months before you strain it. To strain the mix, get some muslin cloth and a pot, and strain the mix through the Muslin. Depending on what herb you are using, you may need to strain it a couple of times. Once strained, decant the liquid into clean sterile bottles, label them, and there you have your tincture.

### 10.22 Poultice

Using a poultice is a good way of using herbs on localized injuries such as sprains, fractures, and aching muscles and joints. To make a poultice you need a handful of leaves, flowers or roughly-chopped dried roots, or a handful of fresh root that has been battered with a stone to release its pulp.

To make a poultice from roots, put the roots in a stocking or pantyhose leg, and tie a knot. Put the bundle into a pan of boiling water and boil for a few minutes. Turn the heat off, and let it cool down in the pan until it has reached a comfortable temperature. Take it out of the pan while still fairly hot, but not too hot to touch, and place it on the affected area (don't empty the pan: you may be reusing the liquid to reheat the poultice).

Wrap a warm towel round the limb and poultice, and let it sit for as long as you can, preferably at least an hour. In the first two days of the injury, once the poultice has cooled down, put it back in the pan, reheat it, and repeat the application. Keep reapplying the poultice through the day, and leave it on through the night.

To make a poultice using fresh leaves, boil the leaves for a couple of minutes, take the mash out, strain it, and spread it on a cloth. Wrap the cloth with the mash around the affected limb, and let it sit for an hour or two (or just leave it on).

Alternatively you can blend up the cooked fresh leaves and spread the blended mash on the cloth before applying to the affected area. Poultices are best used repeatedly through the day for a few days. When I have had hairline fractures that did not need setting, I have used a comfrey poultice many times, and it is amazing how strongly it works.

## 10.23 Summary

Because herbs are often different from country to country, it is pointless for me to go into a detailed list of various herbs that can be used fresh or can be worked with magically (also, I am not a herbalist and I have limited knowledge). If you want to work with living and fresh herbs, it would be a good idea to research your local plants and get a few good old-fashioned herb books.

I have never managed to find a good all-over herb book; instead I have a few different ones that I try to learn from in regards to local medicinal and magical herbs for the land that I live upon. Older ones that concentrate on folk legends and remedies are usually the best, as they are often written from direct experience. All too often these days, herb books—and sadly in particular those books that straddle the line between magic and herbs—are written by people who have not actually used or worked in any depth with the herbs that they write about.

For buying tinctures and medicinal herbs in capsules, there is a wealth of information and suppliers on the net, and the internet gives us the freedom to explore more exotic herbs and medicinal systems like Ayurvedic herbs, Chinese herbs, etc.

Never take anything at face value: all bodies are different, and what works for one person may not work so well for others. Experiment, use readings, and see how your body responds to various substances: at the end of the day, your body knows best.

As for growing herbs, working with them magically, or harvesting them to work with them, it pays to take the time to research what grows naturally in your area, and what it was used for. Look for good organic fertilizers, and watch carefully to see how different plants get on with each other. Some buddy up, some fight, and some overwhelm the more delicate plants around them.

Don't make the obvious mistake of trying to 'organize' your herbs into neat little rows and then weeding them furiously. Let them wander and find their favourite part of the garden, let some weeds grow among them to keep the soil strong and deter pests, and always let at least part of your garden go a bit wild (unclipped) so that the insects, reptiles, and spiders can flourish. They all keep the garden in balance and healthy. Long lawns with pretty neat flowers may look good, but it is a nature desert.

Another very magical act when growing herbs is to grow plants not just for yourself, but also to plant herbs, bushes and

## 10. Herbs and Substances

flowers for the bees and birds. I plant a lot of flowers and bushes for the various types of bees that live near me, and have berry bushes for the birds. If you have space, make a bee hotel in the garden for them to winter over in, and put up nesting boxes for spring. Have old log piles in corners for insects, reptiles and snakes, as it is their land too. If you are in an area with venomous snakes and spiders, do the pile away from the house, and warn children to stay away from them. Watching a garden flourish and mature is a wonderful thing, as is building a relationship with the land, the plants, and your own body.

Chapter Eleven

# *Approaches to self-healing and maintenance*

## 11.1 Magical, emotional, and physical considerations

Working within magic brings about change; it is as simple as that. How we handle the changes to our lives, our health, our minds, and our spirit determines what harvest we will reap. The longer we operate within magic, the more we become exposed to the complexity of how power, life, and our role within the manifest world all hang together.

Once the fallacy of 'magic gives you what you want' falls away, then we are left staring at ourselves in the mirror, and we begin the long walk towards understanding just how complex, powerful, beautiful, and difficult magic really is. That walk takes a lifetime, and the further down the road we walk, the more we realize just how little we know and how little we can truly control.

## 11.2 Emotional baggage

The dawning of magical awareness brings with it changes to our health as our minds struggle to let go of the unhealthy things that we cling to. The more we let go of our emotional baggage, the more our body engages with the process and attempts to rebalance itself by cleansing itself of emotional and physical toxicity.

Sometimes that rebalancing works, and sometimes the body or mind is too damaged or toxic to achieve such a wondrous goal. We cling to a sense of victimhood, and feel a need for 'justice' to be done in matters both tiny and great, and this clinging to emotional need buries itself within the body's structure and churns silently away until the body is no longer able to hold it.

## 11. Approaches to self-healing and maintenance

When we are badly hurt physically or emotionally by others, it is part of the psychological process to want justice or revenge, and there is nothing wrong with those feelings. Where it becomes a problem for a magician is when those feelings trigger energetic ties that feed back and forth in a continuous cycle.

That energetic structure builds on itself, and becomes an automated loop of emotion that the magician can get badly tangled within. Parasites become attracted to the energy feed, which they see as a free lunch, and the magician becomes caught in an energetic relationship that connects them to their attacker in a constant energy loop upheld by beings that are enjoying the meal.

Walking away from that dynamic is very hard and is best done in increments, depending on just how much emotional damage you have sustained. Turning your focus away from others, and instead investing your energy in healing yourself, moving forward, and getting on with life frees up all of that trapped energy that is rotting within you.

Being able to let go of things is a major ingredient towards maintaining our physical, mental, emotional, and magical health. Someone does terrible things to you, and you want justice. Learning how to let go of that need for justice, and being able to focus upon sorting yourself out regardless of the actions of others, enables your deeper energies to let go of all the threads and connections, and instead focus on moving forward to heal, learn, and grow. This growth is not only emotive or spiritual; it flows deep down into the body as well, teaching each cell how to patch up, move on, and not be dragged back into a cycle of holding, waiting, and festering.

I do not say this lightly, or from a place of theory or ignorance. I have been around for a while now, and have experienced many unpleasant things done to me in my time. The greatest lesson I have drawn from those experiences, some of which were severe, is an understanding that letting go, moving forward, and flowing around the 'punches' frees up the spirit and the body. Only then can the body focus on dealing with the necessary repair, which in turn enables us to engage fully with magic.

For a magician those 'punches' can come hard and fast over a prolonged period of time, simply because of the power dynamic of magic. The more you learn, the more challenges you are presented with, and the more the facades of life fall away to expose a deeper truth.

Regardless of the irreparable damage the body may have in later years, healing and then maintaining ones health starts from within, deep in your spirit centre. And such deep healing comes from letting go.

Only you can do that. No healer, no teacher can be with you in that process: it is something you must do a day at a time, a situation at a time. It cannot be accelerated by meditation or counselling; it is a tactile experience that tiptoes up on you if you are willing and able to see the opportunities that present themselves.

Once you are willing to engage that process consciously, then a path will open up before you that slowly walks you through deeper and deeper octaves of the experience, until the letting go allows your emotive, ego-driven needs to slowly but surely dissipate. That in turn leads you to deeper parts of yourself, and from those depths you are able to access the strength needed to wield magical power.

Letting go of the emotional need for revenge, recognition and justice is not a coward's way out: it takes considerable strength to walk away from such dynamics, and it does not mean that justice will not be served. As you move deeper into magic and begin to learn the power of balance, of the scales of Ma'at, you will slowly see how things have a way of sorting themselves out.

Besides the deeper and more spiritual, emotional aspects of the body's healing mechanism, it is also important to deal with the more surface presentations of *dis-ease*, which we have looked at in depth in this book. In between those two aspects is the maintenance of the body and its energy within the flow of magic, which is what this chapter is about.

## 11.3 Magical maintenance

No checklist or recipe exists for maintaining your health while walking a magical path; magic, power, and the interweaving of those energies with life is not that simple. In truth, there is no 'clearing and cleansing' ritual that will sweep away every nasty from your path on a daily basis when you are a magician working with deeper aspects of power.

Maintaining a healthy spiritual, physical, and environmental balance is simple, and yet profoundly complex. It is the root principle of true magical self development—and the mystery most damaged by psychology. However, some basic principles can help a magician establish a strong, healthy foundation to

## 11. Approaches to self-healing and maintenance

stand upon. Some of the recommendations I am about to make might seem to come from a moralistic standpoint; that would be an incorrect assumption.

Sadly, magical and mystical dynamics and wisdom have long been twisted in their application by unscrupulous, ignorant and manipulative priesthoods within religions. Our vast wealth of magical, spiritual and mystical texts have been constantly rewritten or altered to manipulate and subjugate in line with dogmas and misunderstandings of the deeper mysteries.

Those manipulated 'truths' become moralistic dogma, and any intelligent person can see the emptiness in such falsehoods. As a result, the moral dogma is rejected along with the original dynamics of the mystical truths hidden within the texts. So please bear that in mind when you read the following information. . None of it has anything to do with morals, but it has everything to do with how magical energy works.

### 11.4 Keeping clear of tangles

One of the single biggest drains on a magician and their health is energetic tangles. These tangles are created by magical action, and the more emotional investment is put into the action, the stronger and more complex the tangle becomes. Some of these tangles or links are a necessary side-effect of essential magical work, but many are totally unnecessary and usually counterproductive in the long term. And it is the long-term consequences of magical action that are usually the most overlooked, especially by younger and less experienced magicians.

Any magical action has a short-term, medium-term and long-term effect, both on the target of the magic and on the magician themselves. The long-term effects can also spill out into the local community or family of the magician, and the consequences of this continued ripple of power usually pass unseen by novice magicians. That is why magicians do less and less magic as they learn and mature, but when they do take action it is focused, powerful, and necessary.

Let's have a look at a practical example. Two young magicians clash on some matter (which is a daily occurrence these days). One magician thinks that the other magician is dangerous or 'bad,' and they decide to bind the ritual words, actions, thoughts, and visions of the offending magician. The short-term effect on the magician doing the binding is to be drained from the work, but such an effect is transient. The short-term effect on the victim is to suddenly find him or herself unable to get into vision, or unable to do rituals. They forget rituals, lose tools, or find they cannot get a clear mind to go into vision.

The medium-term effect of this binding on the victim is a slowing-down of their magical and spiritual development: they are not able to do any magic, therefore they are not able to learn from mistakes; they are not able to see the consequences of any action, nor are they able to commune with beings who could steer them onto a more solid path.

In effect, the binding has stunted their spiritual and magical growth. If they persist in trying to continue magical actions despite the bindings, then their immune system will begin to react to the binding and they will become ill. This in turn begins to pull on the energy of the magician who did the binding. The arresting of the spiritual development of another human being has many energetic consequences: it takes a lot of energy to stop a person walking towards Divinity and spiritual development.

Even though that was not the original intent of the magic, it is a direct consequence which draws more and more energy into the process as it unfolds. So the magician who did the binding becomes energy deficient as their resources are drained off. This can go on for some time without being fully noticed if the magician had good energy reserves to begin with: it is only when the pot is almost empty that the body's alarms go off.

So at this point in the story, we have one magician who is spiritually and magically arrested, and another who is in energy deficit. It is very likely that neither of them is aware of the source of their problems. They may limp on like this for years without fully realizing what is happening to them.

The long-term consequences of this type of binding are very sad indeed. For the magician who was bound, it is most likely that their magical and spiritual life will grind to a total standstill. Instead of slowly developing and maturing, the person is almost essentially 'locked' into their body, and yet the spirit will still strive for power, which is the usual emotive catalyst that takes people to magic in the first place.

That striving for power will instead be focused on their everyday life, which can manifest as a constant attempt to exert control over the people closest to them. This is not a good dynamic, and it often creates egomaniac manipulative control freaks who make other people's lives a misery.

This scenario does not tend to happen if the initial catalyst for

## 11. Approaches to self-healing and maintenance

magic in the victim's life was a wish to commune with Divinity. In such cases the communion will still happen in a limited way, even though they are magically bound, but such a dynamic will often cause profound suffering in their body.

On the other end of the seesaw is the magician who did the original binding. A couple of decades or more down the road of life, and the threads of the magician's energy tied up in the binding action are getting heavier and heavier. By doing the binding they 'created' a life-path for their victim. As its 'creator' they are energetically upholding all the threads of action, energy exchange, and the weight of the web pattern of the victim's life.

The fact that the victim did not manage to fulfil their potential spiritual development through experiential learning is one burden to be carried. The suffering of subsequent victims caused as a result of the bound magician turning into an oppressor also becomes an energetic burden: those threads have to be upheld too. You are responsible for the monsters you create.

Let's go back to the beginning of this story to see how magic could and should have been used. The 'when and where' of magic is even more important than the 'how,' but that understanding can often come quite late in a magicians development, as these days magic is often taught from an egocentric point of view. The modern approach to many forms of Western magic is a result of the post-Victorian magicians: it is about ones 'will' and 'control,' which is very much a 'toddlers' perspective, as opposed to 'need' and 'participation.'

Back to the beginning. There is a young magician who is throwing their weight around in an unhealthy way, or so it is perceived by another young magician. The first step is to use divination to look at the long-term consequences for the people, beings and land around the offending magician. If they are simply going to blow themselves up or degenerate down into a pile of shit, then that is their choice and their business: most of the time, these sorts of issues have a way of working themselves out.

If it looks like their actions are going to have severe long-term consequences for others, then the next step would be to look at the situation through divination to ascertain whether or not such disaster is indeed fated and necessary. It is possible that the negative actions of the magician are providing a conduit for the power of Ma'at to flow through, and bring about a balancing of scales. If this is the case, then it is not your place to interfere (remember, destruction lives alongside regeneration and creation). But if it is not a necessity, then it may be wise to act.

The next step, to take necessary magical action without being personally tied to the fate pattern of the person, is to work unconditionally with the angelic beings that pattern the future. That means you act as a human catalyst for whatever is necessary to bring about a healthier pattern to the situation. That might indeed mean the 'bad' magician is blocked from magic, or that they drop dead, or that they cross paths with someone who changes them, or that they have an experience that changes their life and therefore their magic.

Another, more conditional form of magic that could be appropriate to use under certain circumstances (though not all, so check through divination first) is to indeed bind the magician, but use your words and intent carefully and specifically: bind them only from using magic that specifically hurts other humans and beings. This still carries some energetic tangles with it, but not many. It will not arrest the other magician's potential for development, but it will stop them using magic to kill, rape, or destroy others.

Taking this approach requires the magician who instigates the action to be removed from any ego-driven agenda or emotive action. If the magician feels that 'they are right', that is their ego talking. If they want the person out of their life because the bad magician is an annoyance, then their ego is sitting in the magical driving seat. The variables are many, but you get the idea. Which takes us back to the earlier conversation in this chapter about being able to step away from emotional and ego-driven wants and needs: hopefully now you can see the immense tangles that magicians can become caught up in.

## 11.5 Everything has its own time for resolution

Before I plough into paragraphs about how to maintain the physical and emotive body, there is one more thing that would be useful for a magician to know and understand in regards to managing their health. And that is the dynamic of timing.

Everything that magic touches has its own 'time.' It is a really interesting dynamic, whereby any energetic magical process that has been set into motion already has its time of resolution patterned into the process. What this means for a magician is that healing will come at the right time, in the right place—and

## 11. Approaches to self-healing and maintenance

not before. This is important to keep in mind when you are trying to bring healing to a body, specifically when that body is involved with magic. The same dynamic also works for major magical projects.

So for example, say a magician has been undertaking a long, drawn-out series of magical workings, and his body has also been struggling with illness. Everything that the magician has done to try and bring healing, be it vision, herbs, etc. has only worked up to a point. The magician gets to their breaking-point, and feels that they cannot carry the burden any longer, as their body and mind is beginning to collapse under the strain. The magician may feel that their ability to 'divine' a solution is clouded, and that they are thrashing about in the dark.

One day, without warning, the solution appears: the resolution of the suffering and the resolution of the work turn up together. Energy rushes into the magician to patch up the deficit, and suddenly everything moves forward. In retrospect, the magician looks at their astrology chart and sees how there was a particular alignment that was favourable to such a leap forward. Remember that magic is a process: it will not be hurried, but it will not forget you or leave you behind.

### 11.6 Energetic resources

The magical understanding of energy resources and how to manage them is little known about in today's world of magic. To put it in a nutshell, imagine that when you are born you have a series of 'energy pots' that have varying capacities for holding and distributing energy. Some pots are larger than others, and some have a greater carrying capacity than others. These 'pots' are stored within your 'house of life' and are managed by your guardian angel. This is a very simplistic description, but it gives you a general idea of how the dynamic works.

Having an understanding of your accessible resources and using them wisely is of paramount importance in magic, as is learning not to interfere with them—a lesson I learned in an immediate and very harsh way. I learned about these 'pots' from an inner contact while I was working magically in Egypt, and I was fascinated.

I decided to experiment with these pots, to see if I could move resources from one pot to another. The inner contact had shown me my 'house of life,' and I saw that my 'pot of health' was looking very low in its energy capacity, but my 'pot of outer

## 11.6. Energetic resources

resources' (wealth) was more or less unused. I decided to move energy from my 'wealth pot' and put it into my 'health pot'.

The effects were immediate. Suddenly I was filled with energy and was annoying everyone around me by bounding about full of beans: I became super efficient and glowing with health. Two days later I lost my job, and I was suddenly without any income of any kind.

I went in vision to my 'house of life' to talk with my guardian angel. I got a long lecture about human stupidity and short-sightedness, and was forced to reverse the magic that I had done. The angelic being said it was its job to move resources about as necessary, in accordance with long-term patterns within my life and fate.

I did not like that sense of personal inaction, and I asked the angelic being what action I could take to help facilitate the best use of my remaining resources. The angel showed me the various foolish actions I had done in the past which had wasted precious energy. I was also shown how magically taking or asking for energy from other places outside of my own resources could affect my own energy stores: the deficit caused elsewhere would be balanced using my own energy—there was no free lunch.

I worked in vision over a series of weeks to commune with the angelic being to learn as much as I could, and then spent time looking back over periods of my life that the angelic being had identified as times when I had foolishly squandered precious power, and other periods where I had used my power wisely.

I saw that sometimes the creation of a deficit was necessary, and how at those times the other unused resources were shared out to compensate. This in turn led me to look at magical energetic dynamics in a different way, and to understand just how complex magical actions can really be.

It also showed me how some magicians have 'deeper pockets' than others in terms of resources to draw on, and that such dynamics are personal to you and cannot be compared to others. Each magician is born with the potential resources they need in order to achieve whatever it is they need to achieve. Whether they are successful or not depends on how they approach life, what they do magically, and how their decisions affect the balance of their resources.

Squandering resources creates a deficit, while hoarding them stunts magician magician's inner growth: neither is helpful and the way forward is somewhere in the middle. The first important step is to find out which resources you have in abundance, and

## 11. Approaches to self-healing and maintenance

of which ones precious little remains. . Learning how to use them wisely is the second step. Where we have an abundance of resources we can share, help others, and use them in long-term service. The resources we have precious little of we must protect and use wisely.

By sharing our abundant resources, we create a pattern between ourselves, humans, and other beings (and the land, etc.) that supports rather than entangles: we connect into the communal web that is creation. It also lets us tap into the great energetic recycler , which is in effect an energetic web that interconnects us. When we give freely of our energetic wealth when it is needed by others, the web upholds us when we are in deficit: by giving, we receive. This does not happen automatically: first we have to be willing to share our resources as magicians. When we do share, that connects us to this larger energy community, and power flows to and from us as is needful: we become an energetic collective rather than standing alone. This interaction in turn forces us to make connections: we support each other in various ways where there is true need, both consciously and unconsciously, physically and energetically. What this collective will not do, however, is uphold you when you have squandered resources unwisely: first and foremost you must be responsible for your own energy.

To cut a very long story short, the most useful advice is to be aware that all of your resources, be they health, financial, emotive, magical, or prophetic are all limited and should be used wisely. They can be interchangeable, and you are likely to have strong resources in some aspects and weaker ones in others. Recognizing where your weaknesses lie and protecting those areas by not squandering their energy is an important part of keeping your mind and body together in magic. Recognizing where you have a lot of resources is probably your key to where your path of service lies.

These pots of resources can also be affected by bindings placed on you by other magicians in an attempt to limit you, just as your angelic being can limit your access to a good resource until the time when it is truly needed. So it pays to keep an eye on them to ensure they are not being interfered with.

What I took away from this experience is the need to learn how to trust, and also how to be responsible for myself energetically. If you waste a lot of your resources over decades and then cry for more, your cries will be met with a stony silence.

If you try to take more from other places, you will slowly spiral into more and more deficit (think credit card debt).

If, however, you recognize that you have squandered (which we all do at some point, particularly in our youth) and work magically from an understanding that you will now have some limitations, then you will find that between your focus of action and the overseeing of your energy management by your angelic being, you will find ways to operate very efficiently.

Also, if you learn from your youthful mistakes and engage in proper resource management with your guardian angel, and you are committed to long-term magical service of some kind, then you will benefit when necessary from the scale rebalance and the communal web. This usually comes in terms of mundane resources like food, shelter, skills etc. What you do not have will come to you through various outer channels as and when you need it.

Those who have an abundance of resources pass their surfeit on to those in deficit. In turn that resource is used for magical service that benefits the wider future. This is turn weaves a web of communal cooperation and support. The Inner Library is one manifestation of that communal web: it is the communal collection of energetic resources that we use as knowledge.

The visionary image of the house of life and the energy pots is simply an interface that we can use to tap into that energy dynamic. It seems to have been something the ancient Egyptians knew about, and at some point in time I would like to return to Karnak to search for remnants of this mystery in the paintings and architecture. Once you have experienced this visionary interface directly, then you will begin to recognize it in mystery texts.

These limited resources are another reason to think carefully about using magic to get laid, get a car, a healthy bank balance, etc. The powers that flow through magic are profound, and we are inextricably linked into the complex web of energy/power: to squander such precious resources on things that we could achieve for ourselves without magic is a folly and can be a very expensive folly in energetic terms.

## 11.7 Scapegoating

This is another energy dynamic that I have talked about in some of my other books, but here is a brief summary. If you are involved in a magical group, lodge, or organization, then there

## 11. Approaches to self-healing and maintenance

is a possibility that you could be used as a scapegoat for magical rebound. What this means is that your group's leader or leaders can initiate magical actions that would normally result in an energetic backlash on them. To avoid that backlash, the leader magically assigns (usually without the victim's knowledge) a member or members of the group to act as a scapegoat for the backlash. This neophyte not only suffers a loss of energy, but also the energetic consequences of their leader's magical action, while the leader gets off Scot-free.

This does not happen too often, as many magicians these days do not know how to do it. But it does happen, and it is nasty. This can be identified by observing changes to your energy and health when you are involved in a group. If you join a lodge or group and find that you slowly become sick, drained or depressed, and unhealthy things are happening around you, then it is time to use divination to find out if indeed you are being scapegoated.

Such a collapse of your health and life pattern upon joining a lodge can be for a variety of reasons, not just scapegoating, so do not jump to conclusions. Sometimes initiation can throw your life up in the air to rearrange you: you are broken down before being rebuilt.

It can also happen if the group is unhealthy: you begin to get dragged down by the parasites that usually frequent unbalanced lodges. The way to tell what is happening under such circumstances is to use divination(the Tree of Life layout is best for yes/no answers), and clearly ask 'am I being scapegoated?' If the answer is no, then the next question should be, 'is this destruction necessary for my development?

If you find yourself in a scapegoat situation and it is making your body ill, then the magical impact has already embedded itself within your physical structure. The way to remove such embedded bindings is to do a visionary body cleanup, and then take a consecrated ritual bath where you specifically direct the ritual to remove the bindings of the scapegoat.

Keep a close eye on the effects a group is having on you, which in turn will enable you to make more informed decisions about your membership of that group. Part of the overall maintenance of a magician's health and strength is proactive awareness.

## 11.8 Physical maintenance

The best way to keep your body in good (or at least reasonable) health is a basic, old-fashioned common-sense rule that we often forget in today's crazy world. Sunshine is one of the greatest healers, and the sun gives us strength physically and magically. Most often these days we spend a lot of time indoors, and are told that the sun will give us cancer. Too much of anything is bad for you, but where sunshine is concerned we tend to go to the other extreme in avoidance.

As a magician, going out each day for a walk, being in sunlight, greeting the sun, and sitting in its power are some of the most powerful things you can do to uphold your health. You should bathe in the sun, the air, and the nature around you on a daily basis. If that is not possible, perhaps because of work commitments, then do it as often as you can. Exposure to sunlight is not a magic pill to make you better, but it is a major element of healing and maintenance for magicians.

The same goes for eating food that has life in it, and keeping to healthy sleep cycles. If you regularly stay up through most of the night, then do not be surprised if your immune system, heart and central nervous system eventually begin to falter. Resetting and repairs to the body are done at specific times through the night, and daytime sleep does not work in the same way. The body works with tides, with the moon, with the seasons, with day, and with night: we happily pour over tables and correspondences for magic, but few apply the same diligence to their own bodies.

Magic and life are not separate: they are of one another. The repair cycle for your body begins around midnight and continues until dawn. Give your body the sleep that it needs, and don't forget that a lot of magic happens or continues in your sleep.

## 11.9 Getting maintenance work done

In the previous chapters we looked at a couple of healing modalities that a magician can learn and apply to themselves. Sometimes, however, it is needful to go to someone for treatment or to have maintenance work done on your body to keep you on your feet. There are lots of different forms of healing out in the world, and everyone will find one that suits their body best. As always, remember that each body is different,

## 11. Approaches to self-healing and maintenance

and what works well for someone may not necessarily work well for another.

The two main forms that I have found the most helpful for me are acupuncture and cranial osteopathy (not cranial sacral therapy). Both of these healing forms work deep into the body, and access the levels within you that are active in magic. Whichever form of healing you look to, ensure that it has a physical element to it: the treatment needs to ground within the body itself as well as operate within the energetic sphere. Simply manipulating a person's energy through spiritual or energetic healing will not help a magician as much as something that has a physical element to it: magic goes through the whole body from energy to physical substance. Any healing needs to follow those same paths.

When a body is not involved in magic, it is not pliable energetically, so energy healing can truly balance such denseness. But once the body, spirit, and energy of a person has worked within magic and has become looser in its boundaries, then it becomes really important to ensure that any healing form spreads across all aspects of a person.

With acupuncture, once the body has learned how the system works, it can be useful to learn the basic channels and points so that you can manipulate them through finger pressure after magical workings: sometimes a flow of energy becomes stuck or clogs up from the magical impact. The points affected will become sore, and if that happens, rubbing or pressing on them can help to free things up. This is not a replacement for proper treatment, but it helps, particularly if you have no money for a treatment.

### 11.10 Astrology

It can be very useful to learn the basics of how to look at a chart and recognize specific transits that are occurring for you. Rather than plan actions around specific astrological events, it is better to 'go with the flow' and look in retrospect.

Astrology can also be used in maintaining your energy levels within magic, and protecting your health. If your emotional or physical health takes a dive, or your outer life is a bit turbulent, it pays to look at your own chart with transits to see what dynamics are currently at play. Sometimes it is a development process you are going through, and astrology can highlight the specifics for you. Once you know what process is unfolding and what planets are involved, then you can actively engage with the process and with the powers flowing through your life, which in turn enables you to get the most out of the transient powers.

There are a variety of websites that offer free chart drawing, with current transits listed along with explanations. It is a useful learning tool to keep track of your chart, and it also helps you to understand a little bit more about the consciousness that flows through the planets and how they can affect you. It is not necessary to learn astrology in depth, but a rudimentary understanding is very helpful.

## 11.11  Lose the New Age bullshit

This in itself can be a major help when it comes to maintaining your body and spirit. The whole 'New Age' industry makes billions out of telling people what they want to hear, and not what they should hear. This is particularly true in regards to health and energy issues.

We are told repeatedly that if we live as clean spiritual beings, we will never be sick. This is total tosh, and is a shining example of how wisdoms can be twisted into dogmas. This perpetuated lie has caused untold suffering to many people who have been treated as spiritual exiles because they are sick.

Bodies get sick. Bodies get into accidents, have inherited disease, and have stress; the list of what can affect our health is endless. Some sicknesses can be treated medically; others can be treated through alternative medicine and energy healing. Some illnesses and disabilities cannot be fixed, and the magician has to learn how to continue operating within their limitations.

Magicians who innovate and explore are more likely to take constant body hits or end up with chronic illness than those who trot along comfortably in a teaching group. The true key to magical health is about upholding, maintaining, listening to the body, and making the best of what you have.

The other New Age bullshit bullet to dodge is the constant aggressive sale of 'wonder nature cures.' Some are no better than snake oil, but others are true healing substances taken out of context, refined, and made into a supplement that you are told you must take every day (at great expense). Don't get sucked into the bullshit. Learn about your own body, learn about substances and how they work, and do not get trapped in the endless New Age loop of pseudoscience.

## 11. Approaches to self-healing and maintenance

## 11.12 Summary

Keeping your mind and body together in some form of good condition, while going through the trials of magic, is indeed a trial in itself. A major aspect of such maintenance is ensuring that you tend to the magical, energetic, emotive and physical parts of you: all of these aspects of your existence are interwoven and cannot in truth be separated out. One affects the other, and they are all interdependent on each other.

Whenever you are in doubt as to the wisdom of a magical action in relation to your health or energy, and you cannot find a magical reference to guide you, then use your common sense. Relate your experience to an outer paradigm. For example, imagine that you are not in the greatest of health and you want to work magically in vision and ritual with stellar powers. In everyday life, a magical endeavour like that would equate to climbing Everest while you have flu and a health condition. Not the wisest of choices!

Magic will affect your health, and your health will affect your magic. Always keep that in mind, and any magical teacher who tells you that you can do anything you want magically, and that you will have no consequences, is either an idiot or a magical criminal.

Be kind to your body: it carries you faithfully, powerfully, and adapts to the craziest things you feed it, clothe it in, or do with it. If you work with it, even if you make huge and glaring mistakes (as I have), it will adapt and work hard to carry you through life, until the time when the angel of death stands before you.

Appendix A

# The ritual cleansing of a space, room, or house

The contents of this appendix are the rituals for consecrating salt and water in readiness for ritual cleansing, and the cleansing rituals themselves. Do not overuse these rituals; rather it is better to use them only when they are truly needed.

The rituals call upon God (Kether) and Goddess (Malkuth), the utterance/Word and the manifestation/Earth. This is not a religious assignment; rather it is a recognition of Divine power in its polarized form. The holy water can be assigned to the service of Divinity (spoken as 'God') or to the service of the deities (gods and goddesses).

Use the first two fingers of your right hand to point at what you are working on.

Where you see + it means make the sign of an equal-armed cross over whatever you are working on.

## A.1 Recitation for the consecration of salt and water

Have a bowl of water and a bowl of salt. Light a candle, and put the two bowls in front of the candle.

Recite over the bowl of salt while pointing first two fingers:

> I exorcize thee, creature of the earth, by the living God + the holy God + the omnipotent God +, that thou mayest be purified of all evil influence in the name of Adonai, Lord of all angels and men.

Hold the flat of your hand over the salt.

> Creature of the earth, adore thy creator. In the name of God the father + and God the mother + I bless thee and consecrate thee to the service of Divinity.[1]

---
[1] Or 'to the service of the gods and goddesses.'

## A. The ritual cleansing of a space, room, or house

Recite over the bowl of water while pointing first two fingers:

> I exorcize thee, creature of the water, by the living God + the holy God + the omnipotent God +, that thou mayest be purified of all evil influence in the name of Elohim Savaoth lord of all angels and men.

Hold the flat of your hand over the water.

> Creature of the water, adore thy creator. In the name of God the father + and God the mother + I consecrate thee to the service of Divinity.[1]

### A.2 Recitation of pouring

Recite the following before pouring the salt into the water:

> Lord God, father of the heavens above; great Goddess, mother of the earth, grant that this salt will make for health of the body and this water for health of the soul.

Now pour the salt into the water.

> Grant that they may be banished from whence they are used all powers of adversity; every artifice of evil shall be banished into the outer darkness. In thy holy names, Amen.

Once the salt and water are poured together, the mix is ready to cleanse and purify anything it touches.

### A.3 Cleansing a space

Once you have consecrated the salt and water and poured them together, then it is time to use that mix to cleanse a space. If you are doing a house, make sure you do each room individually. If a room has been changed from two rooms to one room, do the original two rooms.

---

[1] Or 'to the service of the gods and goddesses.'

## A.4 Recitation of clearing

Stand in the centre of each room, and with the two first fingers of your right hand trace a triangle in the air while reciting:

> In the Name which is above every other Name, and in the power of the Almighty…

Point to the top of the triangle.

> …and of the Mother…

Point to the bottom right corner of the triangle.

> …and of the holy spirits…

Point to the bottom left corner of the triangle.
Then point to the middle of the triangle:

> …I exorcize all influences and seeds of evil from this room; I exorcize all demons, parasites, thought-forms, golems; I exorcize all spiritual dirt and evil influence; I exorcize all magical spells, utterances, rituals, curses and bindings of fire, water, earth, or air sent by other humans. I cast upon them the spell-chains, and I cast them into the outer darkness where they shall trouble not these Servants of God. I open all gates for the ghosts of those passed, and commend them to walk to the river of death. Amen, Amen Selah.

## A.5 Ritual bath for body cleansing

Have a full bath of water and a bowl full of salt. Consecrate a bowl of salt and then the bath of water using the techniques listed above. Once that is done, do the *recitation of pouring* and then the *recitation of clearing* over the bathwater.

The person needing the cleansing should then get in the bath. They need to immerse themselves completely, or turn face down into the bath for a brief moment, so that the water touches every part of them. Once out of the bath, dry with a clean towel, and put on clean clothing. Put all the removed clothing in the washer and wash as normal, but add a handful of salt to the washing powder.

Appendix B

# *Technique for making a talisman*

This is a silent, simple ritual that also uses visionary techniques and inner contacts. It is a first line of defence from magical attack or impact, or to protect the magician during times of extreme stress or illness. It can also be used to protect a vulnerable person during a dangerous short-term situation. Do not use a talisman all the time, and do not use one for minor issues.

This method of working uses nondenominational ritual, visionary magic and inner contacts to achieve a simple but highly-effective protection barrier. It can be adjusted to work within a specific tradition by using the deities and inner contacts specific to that tradition. Working this way does not use sigils; rather it allows the metal to become the container for the magic, while the contacts connected to the talisman provide the actual protection.

Talismans made using this method run on the energy of the recipient's body, so it is very important to not take them off or they will 'run down' and stop working. Because of this, it is wise to choose a pendant that the recipient is comfortable wearing all the time, and which can be hidden under clothing if necessary.

When the talisman has finished its job, you will need to throw it into a river or bury it. Keeping that in mind, do not spend a fortune on a fancy solid gold pendant or use an heirloom!

## B.1 Setting up

Get a plain metal necklace with no magical quality, i.e. a silver chain with a small stone on it, or a metal shape. Don't use a pendant with any Kabbalistic, magical, religious or New Age images: the plainer the better (a clean slate to work on). Put it in a bowl of dry salt, and leave it there for 24 hours.

You will need five plain white candles, and one long ordinary candle to use as a taper. Place one candle in each of the four directions, and one in the centre. Place the candles on altars if you can, but have nothing on the altars except the candles. If

## B. Technique for making a talisman

this is not possible, place the candles on small plain surfaces (I have used large hardback books with white cloths over them) or place them directly on a clear floor. This is called creating a neutral space. Do not have images ritual objects, etc. on the altars, as these will influence or block the powers that you need to work with.

Take the pendant out of the salt, and place it on the central altar. Ensure doors are locked, phones are switched off, and that nothing can disturb you as you work.

### B.2 Creating the talisman

Light the candle that sits on the central altar. Close you eyes and still your mind. Spend a few minutes in stillness/void meditation before focusing upon the flame using your inner vision. Open your eyes while continuing to use your inner vision. Be aware of your own inner flame getting bigger and as it grows. See yourself reach inside to your centre, and cup a fragment of your inner flame in your right hand. Imagine yourself holding out that fragment of inner flame, and join it with the central candle flame.

Physically pick up the taper, and light the taper candle from the flame that sits on the centre altar. Once the taper is lit, walk a full circle clockwise around the central altar and/or candle, and then process to the east, still working clockwise: physically light the candle in the east. Stand for a moment with your eyes closed and see the flame with your inner vision. As the flame strengthens, imagine a gate behind the flame, and silently ask for help from the inner beings who reside beyond that gate. Wait until you see the gate to the east swing open.

You become aware of an inner contact, being, deity, priest, or priestess standing behind the flame on the threshold of the gate. Acknowledge them silently before backing slowly away. Then you walk to the south quarter, and so on. Repeat the same action of opening the gates in the south, west and north until all the candles are lit and all the contacts are present. Take your time with this part of the ritual: if you need to repeat this action a few times around the circle then that is fine: it will help to build the power up in the room.

Pick up your talisman and start in the east. Go to the altar in the east, and hold the talisman over the flame (without burning it or yourself). Close your eyes and in vision, ask the inner contact in that direction to put into the talisman whatever is needful for your own (or the recipient's) protection, education and health: tell them why you need help. Watch while they touch, hold, breath or put something into the pendant as you hold it over the flame. When they have finished, thank them and step back. Turn to the south and repeat the same action, and then do the same for the west and north quarters.

When you have finished in the north, turn and stand before the central altar. Imagine power streaming down from the stars, and power rising up from the earth: both streams of power meet around and in the centre of the flame. Hold the talisman into the collection of power while asking for help. When you have finished, place the talisman upon the central altar, bow to acknowledge the powers present, and leave the room. The talisman will then go through a short period of 'cooking' as it bathes in the power that has built up in the room. You will feel when it is completed.

When the talisman is completed (which can take anything from five minutes to thirty minutes), go back into the room and circle the central flame before going to stand before the altar in the east.

Thank the contact in the east that helped you, offer to return the service when needed (the contact will appear in your dreams or visions when they need your help) and watch as they withdraw. The gates will close and upon their closing, blow out the candle and step back. Repeat the same action in the south, west and north, but leave the central candle burning with the talisman upon the altar.

Go and take a ritual salt bath immediately (or if the talisman is for someone else, put them in a ritual bath), and then put the necklace on yourself or the recipient. Close down the contact in the centre using the same methods you worked with in the four directions: see the two streams of power withdraw, and upon that withdrawal, blow out the candle.

## B.3  Maintenance

Don't take the talisman off, even for a shower. It will have a limited lifespan and you will know when it has finished its job as you will either feel the shift, or it will break and fall off. They are meant to provide only short-term protection, so don't overuse them or you will not gain your own inner protection.

## B. Technique for making a talisman

If the talisman takes a hit (breaks, explodes, refuses to stay on) then it is time to take it off and bury it or drop it into a river. Do not be tempted to keep it and reuse it.

Keep the candles in a special place, and only use them for your magical work: the resonance of the contacts will be embedded within the candle wax.

Appendix C

# *Tarot key words for health readings*

## C. Tarot key words for health readings

### C.1 The Minor Arcana

Remember, the court cards can represent different things: powers or people. Sometimes, a king or queen will represent a man or woman of the appropriate astrological sign. For example, the King of Wands can represent a man who has a fire sign rising.

**Swords: Air, force, misfortune, intellect**

| | |
|---|---|
| Ace of Swords | defending, battle, declaration |
| Two of Swords | truce, balance, stasis |
| Three of Swords | separation |
| Four of Swords | sickness, withdrawal |
| Five of Swords | Argument, breathing issues |
| Six of Swords | moving on, fading away |
| Seven of Swords | hidden action, dodging |
| Eight of Swords | trapped, bound |
| Nine of Swords | Suffering |
| Ten of Swords | failure, defeat, crisis |
| Page of Swords | sneaky communication |
| Knight of Swords | a fight, battling infection |
| Queen of Swords | disciplined female power |
| King of Swords | guardian, a warning |

**Pentacles: Substance**

| | |
|---|---|
| Ace of Pentacles | blockage, shield, substance |
| Two of Pentacles | balance (in substance) |
| Three of Pentacles | work or something working |
| Four of Pentacles | clinging to or holding substance |
| Five of Pentacles | not enough resources |
| Six of Pentacles | generosity, access to needful substance |
| Seven of Pentacles | Normal function |
| Eight of Pentacles | skilled application, repair work ongoing |
| Nine of Pentacles | wellbeing, properly-resourced |
| Ten of Pentacles | too much substance, overgrowth |
| Page of Pentacles | child, small growth, parasite |
| Knight of Pentacles | ancestral patterns i.e. genetic illness |
| Queen of Pentacles | older female power, menopause |
| King of Pentacles | ancestor |

## C.1. The Minor Arcana

### Wands: Fire, energy, creativity

| | |
|---|---|
| Ace of Wands | internal fire, energy, the start of something |
| Two of Wands | assessment, watchfulness |
| Three of Wands | activity |
| Four of Wands | happiness |
| Five of Wands | challenge, confrontation, like an infection |
| Six of Wands | victory |
| Seven of Wands | courage, strength |
| Eight of Wands | a lot of energy (can be good or bad, like in a fever.) |
| Nine of Wands | surviving something, overcoming |
| Ten of Wands | Burden, height of fever |
| Page of Wands | enthusiasm |
| Knight of Wands | aggressive/fiery being or illness (e.g. a virus), fire energy |
| Queen of Wands | creative female power |
| King of Wands | aggressive male power (can be good or bad) |

### Cups: Water, fluids, emotions, fertility, beauty

| | |
|---|---|
| Ace of Cups | fluid |
| Two of Cups | balance of fluids |
| Three of Cups | wellbeing (particularly in respect to fluids, e.g. heart, kidneys) |
| Four of Cups | taking in something (e.g. medicine) |
| Five of Cups | fluid imbalance |
| Six of Cups | nurturing, being nurtured |
| Seven of Cups | unseen element, looking in the wrong place |
| Eight of Cups | moving on emotionally |
| Nine of Cups | fluid, emotional stability |
| Ten of Cups | emotional, too much fluid |
| Page of Cups | being offered medicine |
| Knight of Cups | a lover, an assistant |
| Queen of Cups | passive female power |
| King of Cups | passive male power |

## C. Tarot key words for health readings

### C.2 The Major Arcana: the trump cards

| 0  | The Fool             | folly, madness, empty, lacking resources |
| 1  | The Magician         | taking action, a doctor, surgeon |
| 2  | The High Priestess   | using skill and knowledge |
| 3  | The Empress          | creative female power, oestrogen, goddess power |
| 4  | The Emperor          | male power, testosterone, god power |
| 5  | The Hierophant       | spiritual centeredness, intentional celibacy |
| 6  | The Lovers           | union, sex, cooperation |
| 7  | The Chariot          | moving, travel, action |
| 8  | Strength             | literally strength |
| 9  | The Hermit           | introspection, falling back on own resources |
| 10 | The Wheel of Fortune | change |
| 11 | Justice              | harmony, balance |
| 12 | The Hanged Man       | self-sacrifice, service |
| 13 | Death                | transformation, complete ending |
| 14 | Temperance           | being tempered, being protected |
| 15 | The Devil            | imbalance, infestation, disease |
| 16 | The Tower            | destruction (often sudden) |
| 17 | The Star             | new beginnings, nervous system re-firing |
| 18 | The Moon             | illusions, something unseen, mental illness |
| 19 | The Sun              | vitality |
| 20 | Judgement            | a decision |
| 21 | The World            | fulfilment, life |

Bear in mind that these are simple key words and reductions of wider interpretations, so you have to put them in context. The more confident you get with the key words, the more you can begin to explore the deeper meanings of the cards. So for example, in a health reading, the Ten of Pentacles would mean cancer or obesity (too much earth), and the Devil would mean a major infection (trump card, imbalance or invasion).

# Quareia
## A New, Free School of Magic
## For The 21st Century

*Advancing education in Mystical Magic
and the Western Esoteric Mysteries.*

www.quareia.com
schooldirector@quareia.com

Quareia is a practical magical training course founded by Josephine McCarthy and Frater Acher. It is a complete and freely available course designed to develop a student from a complete beginner into an adept. There are no barriers to entry: the course is accessible regardless of income, race, gender, religion, or spiritual beliefs.

Quareia is aligned to no particular school or specific religious, mystical, or magical system; rather it looks at and works with various magical, religious, and mystical practices that have influenced magical thinking in the Near Eastern and Western world from the early Bronze Age to the present day.

The entire course is free and openly available on the Quareia website.

www.ingramcontent.com/pod-product-compliance
Lightning Source LLC
Chambersburg PA
CBHW071730080526
44588CB00013B/1967